LIPPINCOTT'S ESSENTIALS FOR NURSING ASSISTANTS

A Humanistic Approach to Caregiving

Third Edition

Pamela J. Carter, RN, BSN, MEd., CNOR
Program Coordinator/Instructor
School of Health Professions
Davis Applied Technology College
Kaysville, Utah

 Wolters Kluwer | Lippincott Williams & Wilkins
Health

Philadelphia • Baltimore • New York • London
Buenos Aires • Hong Kong • Sydney • Tokyo

Acquisitions Editor: Elizabeth Nieginski/Chris Richardson
Product Manager: Eric Van Osten/Katherine Burland
Project Manager: Priscilla Crater
Editorial Assistant: Zack Shapiro
Design Coordinator: Holly McLaughlin
Manufacturing Coordinator: Karin Duffield
Prepress Vendor: SPi Global

3rd edition

9 8 7 6 5 4 3 2 1

Printed in China

Library of Congress Cataloging-in-Publication Data
Carter, Pamela J.
   Lippincott's essentials for nursing assistants: a humanistic approach to caregiving / Pamela J. Carter. — 3rd ed.
      p. ; cm.
   Essentials for nursing assistants
   Includes index.
   ISBN 978-1-60913-750-2
 I. Title. II. Title: Essentials for nursing assistants.
   [DNLM: 1. Nurses' Aides. 2. Nursing Care—methods. WY 193]
   610.7306'98—dc23
                                                                            2012031982

To all of the instructors who teach Nursing Assisting. You give so much of yourselves to your students. Not only do you introduce them to the health care profession—you mentor them, guide them, and inspire them to become the future of humanistic care.

ABOUT THE AUTHOR

Pamela Carter is a registered nurse and an award-winning teacher. After receiving her bachelor's degree in nursing from the University of Alabama in Huntsville, Pamela immediately began a career as a perioperative nurse. Over the course of her nursing career, she also worked in a physician's office and as a staff nurse in an intensive care unit.

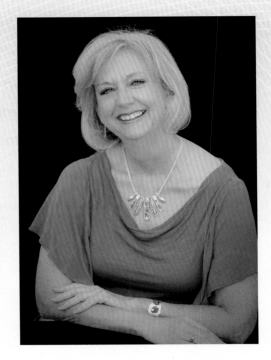

Pamela started teaching informally while serving as an officer in the United States Air Force Nurse Corps. She formally entered the field of health care education by accepting a position at the Athens Area Technical Institute in Athens, Georgia, where she taught surgical technology. After obtaining a master's degree in adult vocational education from the University of Georgia, Pamela moved to Florida and took a position teaching nursing assisting students. She continued teaching nursing assisting after accepting a position at Davis Applied Technology College in Kaysville, Utah. During her first year at Davis Applied Technology College, Pamela piloted a new "open-entry/open-exit" method of curriculum delivery for the nursing assistant program at the college and was awarded the Superintendent's Award for Outstanding Faculty for her work. She then opened a surgical technology program at the college and has obtained national accreditation from the Commission on Accreditation of Allied Health Education Programs (CAAHEP) for delivery of this program using the "open-entry/open-exit" method. In 2002, Pamela received a National Merit Award for having her program rank in the top 10% in the nation for students passing their national certification exam.

In addition to authoring this textbook, Pamela has also authored *Lippincott's Textbook for Nursing Assistants*, "*Lippincott's Textbook for Long-Term Care Nursing Assistants*," as well as *Lippincott's Advanced Skills for Nursing Assistants*. Pamela's writing style reflects her love of teaching, and of nursing. She is grateful for the opportunity teaching and writing have afforded her to share her experience and knowledge with those just entering the health care profession, and to help those who are new to the profession to see how they can have a profound effect on the lives of others.

Nursing assistants are increasingly being hired by health care facilities of all types as these facilities seek ways to provide top-quality nursing care in the most efficient manner. As a result, the need for qualified, well-trained nursing assistants is growing rapidly. Programs that train nursing assistants are tasked with preparing competent workers to meet this growing need as quickly as possible. Different regions of the United States have different requirements that govern the training of nursing assistants. Although different in the depth of training and the number of hours required, all nursing assistant educational programs must meet the minimum requirements established by the Omnibus Budget Reconciliation Act (OBRA) for the number of hours and specific areas of curriculum taught. Many nursing assistant educational programs focus on providing the student with the foundational concepts and facts that he or she will need to function competently in the workplace, whether that workplace is a long-term care facility, hospital, acute or extended care facility, hospice agency, or home health care agency. These *essential* requirements are the focus of this book.

Nursing assistant education is required to focus on skill competency. However, instilling in a new nursing assistant the confidence that he or she can perform the required skills properly is hardly enough. To function effectively in the health care setting, nursing assistants must also be able to recognize the person within the patient, resident, or client, and to understand that each person they are responsible for providing care for is unique and special, with individual needs that are very different from those of the person in the next bed. This textbook, *Lippincott's Essentials for Nursing Assistants*, has been written not only to help students become competent in performing the skills that are the basis of the daily care they provide, but also to teach students to provide that care with compassion and humanism.

GUIDING PRINCIPLES

Three key beliefs guided the writing of this textbook:

1. Students need a textbook that provides foundational concepts and facts in a manner that is easy to comprehend and interesting to read.
2. Graduates of nursing assistant training programs must be able to provide competent, skilled care in a compassionate way.
3. The nursing assistant is a vital member of the health care team.

These beliefs form the basis for the textbook you hold in your hands.

Lippincott's Essentials for Nursing Assistants, 3e, Is Written With the Student in Mind

Educators know that a student can easily understand complex information if it is explained in a way that the student can understand. I have worked hard to develop a conversational, yet professional, writing style that respects the student's intelligence. Concepts are presented in a straightforward, accessible way. Only the most basic, essential information is included, with the understanding that this foundational knowledge will be supplemented by classroom instruction and on-the-job training.

The structure of each chapter helps students in fast-paced, shorter nursing assistant programs learn and retain the information in the chapter. Each chapter is broken down into major sections, each with its own learning objectives (**"What Will You Learn?"**), vocabulary, and summary (**"Putting It All Together"**). This approach allows the student to break up the reading assignment into smaller, more manageable parts.

Vocabulary words are highlighted in the text and defined in the margin. Illustrations are used as necessary to enhance and support the definitions.

Numerous photographs, both alone and in combination with line art, help the student to visualize and remember important concepts. Graphic elements, such as boxes and tables (many of which are illustrated), add visual interest and help to break up the monotony of large expanses of text.

Although the page count makes one think that this text is not short or concise, pages are set up in a "one column" writing format so that information is spread out. The rationale behind this format style is to make the printed information look less intimidating to the student and easier to read and absorb.

New to this Edition!

The profession of health care changes constantly, and as such, information provided in a textbook must also be constantly updated. Each chapter of this text was carefully reviewed and updated according to changes in the health care industry and the needs expressed by instructors and students who use our texts. Some of the changes were simple and are reflected by subtle rewording of information throughout the text. Others were more complex and have resulted in the addition of a few new chapters and features. Updated information new to this edition is summarized as follows:

■ Updates recommended by the Centers for Disease Control and Prevention (CDC) that relate to new infection control guidelines are found in Chapter 10.

■ Enhancement of information related to the involvement of the patient's/resident's family members, in regard to how care is planned and provided, is found in Chapter 5.

■ Updated information about the function of the Joint Commission and Nursing Home Surveys has been added to Chapter 1 to give students a better understanding of how facilities are accredited and monitored as to the quality of care given to patients and resident.

- Information related to mental health has been updated and the topics of post-traumatic stress disorder (PTSD) and substance abuse have been added.

- Information that describes the different phases of rehabilitation has been added to Chapter 9, along with additional information about the role of the nursing assistant in the rehabilitative effort.

- Ergonomics and Workplace Violence are addressed in regard to workplace safety issues in Chapter 11.

- Chapter 13 has been updated to include the revisions made in the 2010 American Heart Association's (AHA's) Guidelines for BLS.

- The updated 2010 Dietary Guidelines for Americans, including the MyPlate information, have been added to Chapter 21. This chapter also includes updated information on Special Diets and information regarding thickened liquids.

- A new chapter has been added to Unit 5 in this edition. Chapter 31, Caring for People in the Home Environment, introduces the student to the roles and responsibilities required of the Home Health Aide.

- All procedures have been reviewed and updated as needed. The addition of a "What You Document" section at the end of each procedure will help remind the student to document care that has been given and increase awareness of observations specific to each procedure that are important to note.

Lippincott's Essentials for Nursing Assistants, 3e, Helps Prepare Students for Clinical Practice

It is my desire to help prepare students to enter the health care profession with the knowledge, skills, and confidence that education and training can provide. In addition, I want to help students develop the compassion and the critical thinking and communication skills they need to function effectively in the health care setting. Several of the textbook's features were designed specifically with these goals in mind:

- **Procedure boxes.** Certainly, a major objective of any nursing assistant training course is to ensure that graduates are able to provide care in a safe and correct manner. Seventy-one core procedures are presented in this text, including all 25 National Nurse Aide Assessment Program (NNAAP) procedures. The procedure boxes provide step-by-step instructions using clear and concise language. Each procedure box begins with a "Why You Do It" statement, to help students understand the "why behind the what," an understanding that is the foundation for the development of critical thinking skills. The concepts of privacy, safety, infection control, comfort, and communication are emphasized consistently in every procedure. Photographs and illustrations are included within the box as necessary. "Getting Ready" and "Finishing Up" steps are included in each procedure. A "What You Document" section is included at the end of each procedure to remind students to document care that has been given. Icons are used to alert students to procedures that are demonstrated on the accompanying video series. To maintain the flow of the text and decrease the "choppiness" that often results from the inclusion of lengthy boxes within the narrative itself, the procedure boxes are referred to in the narrative but grouped together at the end of each chapter.

Procedure Box: Step-by-step instructions for key nursing assistant actions.

PROCEDURE 20-6
Combing a Person's Hair

Why you do it: Combing the hair helps to prevent tangles and gives the hair a neat appearance.

Getting Ready WGKIEPS

1. Complete the "Getting Ready" steps.

Supplies

- paper towels
- wide-toothed comb or pick
- brush
- mirror
- hair accessories (optional)
- detangler or leave-in conditioner (optional)
- towels

Procedure

2. Make sure that the bed is positioned at a comfortable working height (to promote good body mechanics) and that the wheels are locked.
3. Cover the over-bed table with paper towels. Place the hair care supplies and clean linens on the over-bed table.
4. Raise the head of the bed as tolerated. Gently lift the person's head and shoulders and cover the pillow with a towel. Drape another towel across the person's back and shoulders.
5. If the side rails are in use, lower the side rail on the working side of the bed. The side rail on the opposite side of the bed should remain up.
6. If the hair is tangled, work on the tangles first. Put a small amount of detangler or leave-in conditioner on the tangled hair. Begin at the ends of the hair and work toward the scalp. Hold the lock of hair just above the tangle (closest to the scalp) and use the wide-tooth comb to gently work through the tangle.
7. Using the brush and working with one 2-inch section at a time, gently brush the hair, moving from the roots of the hair toward the ends.

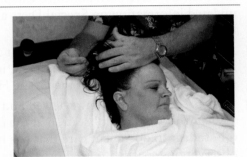

STEP 7 ■ Hold the lock of hair just above the tangle.

8. Secure the hair using barrettes, clips, or pins or braid the hair, as the person requests. Offer the person the mirror to check her appearance when you are finished. Remove the towels from the person's shoulders and the pillow.
9. Reposition the pillow under the person's head and straighten the bed linens. If the side rails are in use, return the side rails to the raised position. Lower the head of the bed as the person requests.
10. Gather the soiled linens and place them in the linen hamper or linen bag. Dispose of disposable items in a facility-approved waste container. Clean equipment and return it to the storage area.

Finishing Up CLSOWR

11. Complete the "Finishing Up" steps.

What You Document

- Date and time
- Type of care provided
- Presence of excessive tangling or any unusual observations of the hair or scalp

- **Guidelines ("What You Do/Why You Do It") boxes.** These boxes summarize guidelines for carrying out key nursing assistant actions. The unique "What You Do/Why You Do It" format helps students to understand why things are done a certain way. I believe that if students understand why something is done a certain way, they will be more likely to remember to do it that way.

Guidelines Box 10-2   Guidelines for Using Gloves

What you do	Why you do it
If the glove tears when you are putting it on, discard it.	A glove that has a hole or tear will not protect your hands from contamination.
Choose gloves that fit properly.	Gloves that are too tight are uncomfortable and may tear. Gloves that are too loose will not stay on your hands.
Use gloves made from another material if you or the person you are caring for is sensitive to latex.	Depending on the severity of the allergy, exposure to latex can cause redness and cracking of the skin, a severe rash, or problems breathing.
Remove contaminated gloves before touching any other surface. You may need to change gloves several times during one procedure.	Replacing your gloves when they become contaminated prevents the transfer of pathogens from dirty areas to clean areas. If you touch a surface (such as the side rail, light switch, or doorknob) with your contaminated gloves, the pathogens will be transferred from your gloves to that surface. The next person who touches the surface could then pick up the pathogens you left there with your contaminated gloves.
Wash your hands after removing gloves.	Gloves are easily torn or may have holes too small to see, causing your hands to become contaminated. Handwashing removes any microbes that may be on your hands.

Guidelines Box ("What You Do/Why You Do It"): Guidelines and rationales for key nursing assistant actions.

TELL THE NURSE !

SIGNS OF INFECTION

- Fever
- A rapid pulse, a rapid respiratory rate, or changes in blood pressure
- Pain or difficulty breathing
- Redness, swelling, or pain
- Foul-smelling or cloudy urine
- Pain or difficulty urinating
- Diarrhea or foul-smelling feces
- Nausea or vomiting
- Lack of appetite
- Skin rashes
- Fatigue
- Increased confusion or disorientation
- Any unusual discharge or drainage from the body

- **Tell the Nurse! notes.** A recurrent theme throughout the book is the important role the nursing assistant plays in making observations about the patient's or resident's condition and reporting these observations to the nurse. The *Tell the Nurse!* notes highlight and summarize signs and symptoms that a nursing assistant may observe that should be reported to the nurse. This information is presented within a context to help students remember and apply the information.

- **Stop and Think! scenarios.** Each chapter concludes with one or more *Stop and Think!* scenarios. These scenarios encourage students to critically solve problems, and help them to see that many situations they will encounter in the workplace do not have cut-and-dried answers.

Tell the Nurse! Note: Observations that need to be reported to the nurse.

 Stop **and** Think!

Mr. Lovell, one of the residents with dementia at the long-term care facility where you work, has become very agitated. He is prone to falling, and should not get up without help. However, today he is refusing to stay in his bed or his wheelchair. You get him situated, and then as soon as you leave the room, he tries to get up again. This has happened twice, and you are only in the first hour of your shift. You are very concerned that Mr. Lovell will fall and hurt himself, but you cannot stay with him all day because you have other residents to attend to. Describe some things that you could do to help protect Mr. Lovell.

Stop and Think! Scenario: Situations to promote critical thinking.

■ **Nurse Pam.** Nurse Pam, modeled and named after the author of this book, appears throughout the text in various scenarios to help students empathize with their patients or residents.

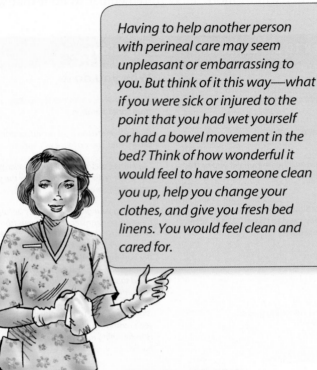

Having to help another person with perineal care may seem unpleasant or embarrassing to you. But think of it this way—what if you were sick or injured to the point that you had wet yourself or had a bowel movement in the bed? Think of how wonderful it would feel to have someone clean you up, help you change your clothes, and give you fresh bed linens. You would feel clean and cared for.

Nurse Pam: Highlights humanistic, holistic care.

Lippincott's Essentials for Nursing Assistants, 3e, Promotes Pride in the Profession

It is my desire to impress upon students entering the health care profession that no one is "just" a nursing assistant. Nursing assistants are often the members of the health care team with the most day-to-day contact with patients, residents, and clients. As such, they bear a large part of the responsibility for the well-being of those in their care. Nursing assistants who feel that they can and do make a difference in the lives of others will go the "extra mile" to ensure that the care they provide is holistic.

AN OVERVIEW OF *LIPPINCOTT'S ESSENTIALS FOR NURSING ASSISTANTS, 3e*

This textbook consists of five units. The following is a brief survey of these units and the information they contain.

Unit 1: Introduction to Health Care

The six chapters that make up Unit 1 provide the student with basic background knowledge. Chapter 1 introduces the student to the health care setting and the governmental regulations that play a role in establishing standards and funding for health care. The nursing home survey process is introduced so that students become better informed of how regulatory organizations determine a facility's ability to provide quality care to the residents. Chapter 1 also introduces the holistic approach to health care. Chapter 2 focuses on the nursing assistant's responsibilities as a member of the health care team. The concepts of delegation and the nursing process are introduced. In addition, Chapter 2 explores legal and ethical issues related to the nursing assistant's job, including patient and resident rights, the Health Insurance Portability and Accountability Act (HIPAA), advance directives, and abuse. Professionalism, job-seeking skills, and the concept of work ethic are thoroughly discussed in Chapter 3, introducing students to the idea that a professional attitude promotes respect and is necessary for career advancement. Communication, one of the most essential responsibilities of the nursing assistant, is discussed in Chapter 4. Chapter 5 focuses on the central member of the health care team—the patient, resident, or client. This chapter introduces the concept of human needs and explains how the person being cared for in a health setting has many needs other than those specifically associated with illness or disability. The impact that illness and disability have on a patient's or resident's family members and their need to be involved in the person's plan of care are also addressed. The unit concludes with Chapter 6, which focuses on the person's environment in a health care setting. OBRA requirements related to the physical environment of a long-term care setting are listed and explained. Updated information on staff work areas has been included in this chapter.

Unit 2: The Human Body in Health and Disease

Having a basic understanding of how each of the body's organ systems functions in health is essential to understanding how failure of an organ system to work properly leads to disease and disability. Chapter 7 gives a basic description of the structure and function of each of the body's organ systems. In addition, for each organ system, the effects of the normal aging process on that organ system's function are described. Chapter 8 discusses disorders that frequently create the need for a person to be cared for in a health care setting. Updated information on different disorders and illnesses has been added, including: Muscular Distrophy, care of hip fractures, vascular disorders, Parkinson's disease, coma and persistent vegetative state, management of diabetes mellitus, neurogenic bladder, PTSD, and substance abuse disorders. Rehabilitation and restorative care are discussed in Chapter 9, with an emphasis on the role that the nursing assistant plays in this important aspect of patient and resident care.

Unit 3: Safety

The four chapters in this unit are concerned with measures taken to ensure safety, both for the patient or resident and for the nursing assistant. Chapter 10 covers communicable disease and how the spread of communicable disease is prevented in the health care setting. Updated guidelines from the CDC have been included. Chapter 11 deals with workplace safety, and includes an extensive discussion about the importance of using proper body mechanics and ergonomics to prevent work-related injuries. Information related to workplace violence and tips on how to avoid and remain safe at the workplace has been included. Chapter 12 explores some of the conditions that put patients and residents at risk for injury, followed by a discussion about methods used to prevent accidents from occurring. Information and guidelines to help prevent "entrapment" has been included to update this chapter. This unit concludes with Chapter 13, which contains information related to recognizing emergencies and responding to them. Expanded information on how to recognize the signs of heart attack and stroke has been added. Chapter 13 also includes the updated 2010 AHA Guidelines for BLS and updated procedures for clearing an obstructed airway.

Unit 4: Basic Patient and Resident Care

The eleven chapters in this unit focus on the skills and equipment used to provide basic daily care to people in a health care setting. In Chapter 14, the techniques used to safely assist patients and residents with repositioning and transferring are explained. Chapter 15 discusses the complications that can result from immobility and explains how to safely assist a person in a health care setting with ambulation and exercise. Chapter 16 describes bedmaking skills. Chapter 17 covers vital signs, height, and weight. Because many students find the procedures related to taking vital signs intimidating and difficult to master at first, encouragement and practical tips are included throughout. Chapter 18 covers bathing and routine skin care. Chapter 19 focuses on the prevention and treatment of pressure ulcers and other types of wound care. Chapter 20 covers routine grooming. In Chapter 21, newly updated information about basic nutrition is presented in a factual, useful manner without undue emphasis on specific diets, as these continue to change as research dictates. New information about preparing and serving thickened liquids has been included. Chapters 22 and 23 cover urinary and bowel elimination, respectively. Unit 4 concludes with Chapter 24, which discusses how the nursing assistant helps to promote comfort, including a discussion about the importance of recognizing and reporting signs of pain.

Unit 5: Special Care Concerns

The final unit in this text contains six chapters that cover special care situations that the nursing assistant will most likely encounter during a career in health care. Chapter 25 describes how a person and his or her loved ones cope with a terminal illness and impending death. The care provided to the dying person in the hours leading up to, and following, death is also discussed. In Chapter 26, the student is provided with specific information about how to communicate with, and care for, people with dementia. In Chapter 27, some of the major types of developmental disabilities are reviewed. Chapters 28 and 29 cover the special care needs of people who have cancer and HIV/AIDS, respectively. Chapter 30 discusses the special care required by patients and residents before and after a surgical procedure.

The newly added Chapter 31 introduces the student to the home health care setting. Building on basic knowledge and skills presented in previous units, this chapter explores some of the concerns and issues that are unique to the home health care setting. Chapter 31 provides students with an overview of what home health care is and who might require it, and explores some of the qualities that a person must have to succeed as a home health aide. Specific issues related to safety and infection control within the home are also covered.

Appendices and Glossary

The textbook concludes with two appendices and a comprehensive glossary.

- Appendix A consists of the answers to the **What Did You Learn?** exercises that appear at the end of each chapter.
- Appendix B introduces the student to the language of health care. This discussion about medical terminology is included as an appendix so that it can be introduced at any point during the training course, and referred to frequently. The tables containing common roots, prefixes and suffixes, and abbreviations are in close physical proximity to the glossary for easy and quick reference. Also included in Appendix B is the Joint Commission's "Do Not Use" abbreviations list.
- The glossary is an alphabetical compilation of the vocabulary words from each chapter.

A COMPREHENSIVE PACKAGE FOR TEACHING AND LEARNING

To further facilitate teaching and learning, a carefully designed ancillary package is available. In addition to the usual print resources, multimedia tools have been developed in conjunction with the text.

Resources for Students

- **Student Resources at http://thePoint.lww.com/CarterEssentials3e** include *Watch and Learn!* (a series of video clips that support information given in the text) and *Listen and Learn!* (an interactive glossary that enables students to hear the vocabulary words pronounced, defined, and used in a sentence, and then to quiz themselves using the flashcard feature). In addition, the *Nursing Assistants Make A Difference!* feature allows the student to listen to first-person accounts of how nursing assistants have made a difference in the lives of patients, residents, clients, and family members. Certification-style review questions help students prepare to face exams armed with confidence and knowledge.
- **Workbook to Accompany** *Lippincott's Essentials for Nursing Assistants, 3e.* This illustrated workbook provides the student with a fun and engaging way of reviewing important concepts and vocabulary. Its multiple-choice questions, matching exercises, true-false exercises, word finds, crossword puzzles, coloring and labeling exercises, and other types of active-learning tools will appeal to many different learning styles. The workbook also contains procedure checklists for each procedure in the textbook.

Resources for Instructors

This third edition comes with a collection of ancillary materials designed to help you organize your class, effectively teach the material, and evaluate your students' progress and comprehension. Resources that can be found on the Instructor Resource DVD-ROM and online at *thePoint*—http://thepoint.lww.com/CarterEssentials3e—include:

- **PowerPoint Presentations** and **Guided Lecture Notes**
- Sample **Syllabus**
- **Test Generator** with more than 700 multiple-choice questions
- **Pre-Lecture Quizzes**
- **Assignments, Discussion Topics,** and **Case Studies**
- **Image Bank**
- **Journal Articles**

Additional Resources

- *Lippincott's Video Series for Nursing Assistants.* Procedure-based modules provide step-by-step demonstrations of the core skills that form the basis of the daily care the nursing assistant provides. *Getting Ready and Finishing Up* actions are reviewed on every procedure-based module, and the themes of privacy, safety, infection control, comfort, and communication are emphasized throughout. Four non-procedure–based modules, on the topics of preparing for entry into the workforce, caring for people with dementia, death and dying, and communication and patient and resident rights, are also available.

- **Copper Ridge** *Dementia Care Modules.* Developed by the esteemed Copper Ridge Institute in affiliation with Johns Hopkins University School of Medicine, this two-CD set consists of nine interactive modules designed to teach students how to care for people with dementia. The causes and types of dementia are reviewed, along with dementia-related behaviors and the best way to manage them. Communication and compassion are emphasized throughout. Learning is enhanced through video clips, interactive exercises, and short multiple-choice quizzes at the conclusion of each module.

It is with great pleasure that my colleagues and I introduce these resources to you. One of our primary goals in creating these resources has been to share with those just entering the health care field our sense of excitement about the health care profession, and our commitment to the idea that being a nursing assistant involves much more than just "bedpans and blood pressures." I hope we have succeeded in that goal, and I welcome feedback from our readers.

PAMELA J. CARTER

HOW TO USE THIS BOOK TO PREPARE FOR CLASS AND STUDY

Learning is an active process. You need to read, make notes, and ask questions about anything you are having trouble understanding. Most students who are successful learners take a three-step approach to learning:

Preview

During the *preview* stage of learning, you focus on preparing yourself for class. Most likely, your instructor will give you reading assignments that must be completed before each class. The course *syllabus* that you will receive at the beginning of the course will tell you when each reading assignment must be completed. The reading assignments give you the chance to get a general idea of what is going to be discussed in the next class.

To prepare for class, just read the assignment as if you were reading a novel or a newspaper for enjoyment. During the preview, you do not need to take notes or try to memorize facts—just read through the material to get the "big picture" of the information you are about to learn. Some people find it helpful to read the chapter out loud to themselves (or into a tape recorder, so that they can listen to the chapter again later). Others like to highlight parts of the chapter using a highlighting pen, or make notes in the margin. Learning becomes much easier when you discover what methods work best for you.

To assist you with previewing, each section in each chapter begins with a *What Will You Learn?* section. This section contains a list of specific goals for that

> Welcome! Health care is an exciting, yet demanding, field. During your training course, you will be expected to learn and apply a lot of new information. My name is Pam Carter, and I am the author of the book you hold in your hands. It is my pleasure and my honor to assist you on your journey toward becoming a health care professional. Let me begin by explaining to you a little bit about how you can use this book to prepare for class and study.

What will you learn?

When you are finished with this section, you will be able to:

1. List changes that occur in a person's feet as a result of aging or illness.

2. State observations that you may make when assisting a patient or resident with foot care that should be reported to the nurse.

3. Demonstrate proper technique for assisting with foot care.

 4. Define the word **podiatrist.**

What Will You Learn?: Specific goals for the section.

section, called *learning objectives*. Learning objectives tell you what you will be expected to know or be able to do to demonstrate complete understanding of the material in that section of the chapter. During the preview stage, the learning objectives can be very useful in giving you an overview of the key goals of that section.

The *What Will You Learn?* section also contains a list of the new vocabulary words you will need to learn. The vocabulary words, which appear in **bold type** throughout the chapter, are listed in the order that they appear. The definition of each vocabulary word is found in the margin near where the word appears in the text. The *Listen and Learn!* icon next to the vocabulary words lets you know that you can visit ThePoint to hear the words in each vocabulary list pronounced, defined, and used in a sentence. This is an effective and fun way to preview vocabulary words! Familiarizing yourself with the chapter's vocabulary words before class puts you one step ahead, because when you hear those words in class, they will not sound strange to you, and you may already know what they mean.

As you read the chapter, look for the *Watch and Learn!* icon too. This symbol lets you know that you can visit ThePoint to watch a video clip that supports the information you are reading about.

View

The *viewing* stage is when you get down to business and really work to understand the material. During the classroom lecture or discussion, highlight important points and take notes as you need to. Ask questions about any of the material that you do not fully understand. Remember, there are no "stupid" questions! If you do not fully understand something, you need to speak up so that the instructor can help you. This is your instructor's job.

Review

After class, go back over the notes you took in class, and re-read the chapter in your book. Some students like to read the entire chapter over again. Others just skim the chapter, paying close attention to the topics they still have questions about. Each section in the chapter closes with a short summary called *Putting it All Together!* which repeats and summarizes the key concepts of that section.

When you feel comfortable with your understanding of the material, test yourself! Go back to the learning objectives in the *What Will You Learn?* section at the beginning of each section in the chapter and pretend they are questions. Try to answer them. If you have trouble answering them, then you know that you need to review those sections of the chapter again. You can also test yourself using the *What Did You Learn?* section at the end of each chapter. The answers to the questions in the *What Did You Learn?* section are in Appendix A in the back of the book, so that you can see how well you understood the material

Putting it all together!

- Clean, dry, wrinkle-free linens promote comfort and rest.
- Clean, dry, wrinkle-free linens help to prevent complications, such as pressure ulcers. Dampness contributes to skin breakdown, and wrinkled sheets can cause friction, both of which are factors in the development of pressure ulcers.
- Clean, dry linens are important for odor and infection control.
- Bed linens are changed according to facility policy and as often as necessary to ensure that the patient or resident has a clean, dry, wrinkle-free bed at all times.

Putting It All Together!: A review of key points from the section.

What did you learn?

Multiple Choice

Select the single best answer for each of the following questions.

1. A person with an airway obstruction will usually:
   a. Have a seizure
   b. Vomit
   c. Be able to speak and breathe normally
   d. Clutch at her throat

2. In the Guidelines for BLS, the "C" stands for:
   a. Cardiac
   b. Consciousness
   c. Compressions
   d. Check for bleeding

3. Where do you place your fist while clearing an obstructed airway in a conscious adult?
   a. On the person's back
   b. Above the person's navel
   c. On the person's chest
   d. Below the person's navel

4. If a person is coughing but able to breathe, you should:
   a. Administer oxygen
   b. Use a finger sweep to remove the object that is obstructing the person's airway
   c. Perform abdominal thrusts
   d. Stay with the person and allow him to continue coughing

5. Which is a sign or symptom of shock?
   a. Low blood pressure
   b. A weak, rapid pulse
   c. Cool, clammy, pale skin
   d. All of the above

6. Which of the following actions should you take to assist a person who is having a seizure?
   a. Protect the person's head by placing a pillow underneath it
   b. Clear the area by moving furniture out of the way
   c. Avoid placing anything in the person's mouth
   d. All of the above

7. Which of the following best describes the recovery position?
   a. Positioned on the back
   b. Positioned on the abdomen
   c. Sitting with the head between the knees
   d. Lying on the side

What Did You Learn?: A tool for self-assessment.

you just studied. Again, if you have trouble answering these questions, then you will know that your studying is not quite finished! You may need to read certain parts of the chapter again, or ask your instructor for help.

Try to set aside short periods of time for studying each day. For example, you might study for 30 to 45 minutes, take a break to do other activities or chores, and then come back and study for another 30 to 45 minutes. After 30 to 45 minutes of studying, most people become tired and lose their ability to concentrate. Studying in short bursts will help keep you focused on the material you are trying to learn.

HOW TO PREPARE FOR TESTS

Did you learn the material or not? This is what instructors want to know when they give tests, quizzes, and exams. Not doing well on a test does not mean that you are a failure. It just means that you need to figure out what went wrong, and make an effort to improve the next time. Perhaps you did not study as well as you could have for the test. Or maybe you got so nervous, you forgot everything you learned when it came time to take the test!

The course syllabus will tell you when a test is scheduled to be given, and what material it will cover. Mark these dates on your calendar, so you are not surprised! Preparing for a test should not be a major event. If you use the preview–view–review approach and study each day, when the time comes to prepare for the test, you will be very well prepared. In the days leading up to the test, all you will need to do is review the material that will be covered on the test one more time, by skimming the chapters in the book and reviewing the notes you took in class.

When it comes time to actually take the test, remember the following tips:

- Relax! You have prepared for this test, and you know the answers to these questions!

- Take a deep breath and make sure you read the directions carefully. The directions will tell you whether there is only one correct answer for each question, or whether it is possible for a question to have more than one correct answer.

- Read each question completely and carefully. Many students answer questions incorrectly simply because they are in a hurry and miss important words, like "except" or "not."

- If the question is a multiple-choice question, try to state the answer in your head before looking at the answer choices. Then read each answer choice before choosing the one that best matches the answer you have in your head. This will increase your confidence that the answer you have selected is the correct one.

- After selecting an answer, avoid second-guessing yourself. Research has shown that your first choice is most likely to be correct, if you studied the material well. Sometimes, however, you will come across a question later in the test that makes you realize that you answered an earlier question incorrectly. In this case, when you are sure that you have made a mistake, it is all right to go back and change your answer. But if you do not have a clear idea of what the correct answer is, doubting your first choice will most likely result in changing a correct answer to an incorrect one!

- If you cannot answer a question, go on to the next. Often, another question on the test will jog your memory and help you to remember the answer to the question you skipped earlier. Just remember to go back over your answer sheet before you hand in your test to make sure you have answered all of the questions.

Many people think that the goal of studying is to pass a test. It is true that as you work through your training course, you will have to pass many tests. And most states require people who want to be nursing assistants to pass a certification exam at the end of the training course. But passing the test is a short-term goal. It is more important for you to be able to remember and use the information that you learned during your training course long after you complete the course and pass the certification exam. The people you will be caring for are depending on you to be knowledgeable and good at what you do. They will be trusting you with their health and well-being. Study hard, ask questions, and remember that each and every person you care for throughout your career deserves the same type of competent, compassionate care that you would expect to be given to your own mother, father, spouse, sibling, or child. As a nursing assistant, you will have the chance to have a positive effect on the lives of many people.

Caring for those in need is very important work. Let me be among the first to thank you for your interest in pursuing a career in health care, and to wish you luck on your journey.

Sincerely,

PAM

REVIEWERS

I would like to extend my heartfelt thanks to my fellow instructors across the country who took the time to review the text and provide me with such valuable suggestions for improvement.

Laurel Alfieri
Cincinnati State Technical and Community College
Cincinnati, Ohio

Carol Bell
Mountainland Applied Technology College
Orem, Utah

Sally Christiansen
Waukesha County Technical College
Milwaukee, Wisconsin

Fay Flowers
NexCare Health Care Training Institute
Westland, Michigan

Kathie Hubatch-Babcock
Nicolet Area Technical College
Rhinelander, Wisconsin

Lyn Kruckeberg
South Central College
North Mankato, Minnesota

Patricia Roark
East Tennessee State University
Johnson City, Tennessee

Linda Schneider
Portland Community College
Portland, Oregon

Heidi Shinabargar
Itasca Community College
Grand Rapids, Minnesota

Gail Spivey
Yavapai College
Prescott, Arizona

Sheree Walters
Mt. Hood Community College
Gresham, Oregon

Juanita Wells
Mott Community College
Flint, Michigan

ACKNOWLEDGMENT

The passage of time and growth create the need for change. Change, especially that which affects the health professions, creates the need to constantly revise and update the material that is used to teach students. Thus, the third edition of this textbook and ancillary package has been completed. Change has also been evident in the talent demonstrated by new team members who worked with me to develop this edition of the textbook and ancillaries. I am most appreciative of the years of guidance and assistance given by Elizabeth Nieginski, executive acquisitions editor, dear friend, and mentor. Many thanks are also owed to our new team members, whose expertise and insight are evident in the quality of this project. They are Katherine Burland, product manager, who jumped into this project with both feet midway through; Zack Shapiro, editorial assistant; and Priscilla Crater, production project manager. As always, I want to extend thanks to all of the sales representatives at Lippincott Williams & Wilkins who share my vision and passion and offer such great support to the faculty members who use this text.

CONTENTS

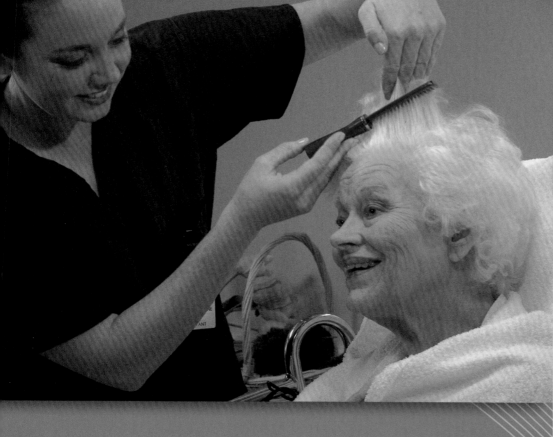

INTRODUCTION TO HEALTH CARE

elcome to the health care field! Today, working in the health care field offers more opportunities than ever before. The health care field is the focus of Unit 1.

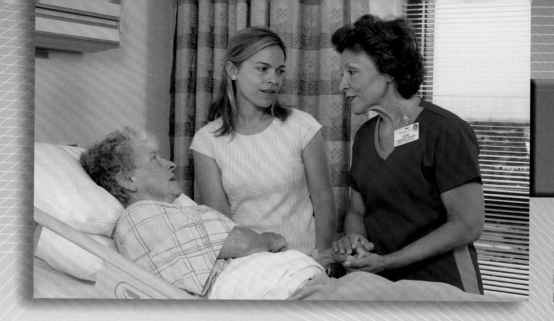

CHAPTER 1

Health care is a people-oriented business.

The Health Care System

As a nursing assistant, you will be part of the health care system. In this chapter, you will learn about how we approach health care delivery in the United States today, as well as about the many different settings in which health care is provided. You will learn about how this system groups people in need of health care. We will also discuss how health care is paid for and some of the government regulations that people working in the health care field need to be aware of.

A HOLISTIC APPROACH TO HEALTH CARE

What will you learn?

When you are finished with this section, you will be able to:

1. Explain how a holistic approach to health care benefits the person receiving care.
2. Explain how the health care team works together to provide holistic care.

3. Define the words holistic and health care team.

In the past in the United States, health care delivery focused mainly around the home and family. Most health care was provided by a family doctor, who would come to the person's home (Fig. 1-1). Because people did not move much and towns were small, the family doctor would get to know each of his or her patients well. The family doctor took care of all of the person's health care needs: for example, he would deliver the babies, attend to wounds and broken bones, and provide comfort to both the dying person and the family.

By the 1940s, this started to change. New medications were being discovered, and new equipment was being developed. Hospitals were becoming more modern. Now, instead of being cared for in their homes, people would go to the hospital when they were sick. As researchers learned more about what causes disease and how to treat it, health care became more complex. Slowly, the family doctor who took care of all of a person's health care needs began to be replaced by a team of doctors, each with a specific type of knowledge.

> *Providing holistic care means recognizing that each person you care for is unique and special, with individual needs that are very different from those of the person in the next bed. While you carry out your daily duties, you will have plenty of chances to get to know your patients or residents as individuals. You will help to take care of your patients' or residents' emotional needs, as well as their physical ones. This is the essence of holistic care.*

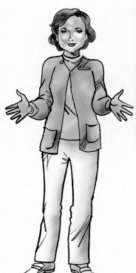

Although the advances in knowledge and technology helped people to live longer lives, an interesting thing started to happen. The focus started to shift from the patient to the technology—from *caring* to *curing*. Fortunately, we are now seeing a return to a more holistic approach to health care. The best aspect of the care provided by the old-fashioned "family doctor"—the doctor's familiarity with the person as an individual—is combined with modern-day availability of specialized care when needed.

Today, holistic care is provided by a health care team made up of many people with different types of knowledge and skill levels (Fig. 1-2). The person receiving the care is always the focus of the health care team's efforts. As a nursing assistant, you will be a member of this team. The job of each member of the team is as important as that of any other member. Think of the members of the health care team as links in the chain of care. Because a chain is only as strong as its weakest link, each member of the health care team must provide care to the best of his or her ability.

Holistic ▪▪▪ care of the whole person, physically and emotionally

Health care team ▪▪▪ group of people with different types of knowledge and skill levels who work together to provide holistic care to the patient or resident

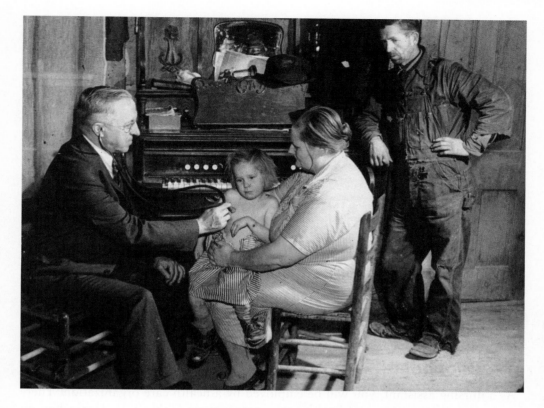

FIGURE ▪ 1-1

In the past, health care was delivered in the home, usually by a "family doctor."

Hafton/Archive by Getty Images.

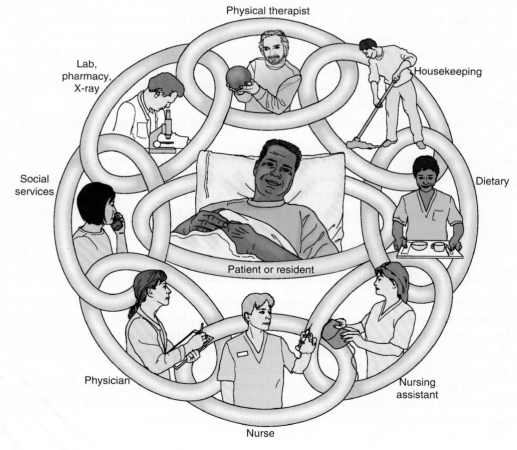

Physical therapist

Lab, pharmacy, X-ray

Housekeeping

Social services

Dietary

Patient or resident

Physician

Nursing assistant

Nurse

FIGURE ▪ 1-2

Care is provided by the health care team. The patient or resident is the primary focus of the team's efforts. Because a chain is only as strong as its weakest link, each member of the health care team must provide care to the best of his or her ability.

Putting it all together!

- Today, we take a holistic approach to health care. That is, we take into consideration the person's emotional as well as physical needs.
- Health care is provided by a team of people, each with different areas of expertise and job responsibilities. The patient or resident is the focus of the health care team's efforts.
- As a nursing assistant, you are a critical part of the health care team.

HEALTH CARE ORGANIZATIONS

What will you learn?

When you are finished with this section, you will be able to:

1. Describe the different types of health care organizations.
2. Briefly explain the structure of a health care organization.

Types of health care organizations

As a nursing assistant, you will be employed by a health care organization. There are many different types of health care organizations (Table 1-1). Depending on where you live, you may be able to work as a nursing assistant in all of these organizations or just some. For example, in some states, nursing assistants are only employed in long-term care facilities (nursing homes), but in other states, nursing assistants can work in hospitals.

Different words are used to refer to people who receive health care, depending on where that health care is provided:

- The word *patient* is used to describe a person who is being cared for in a hospital.
- The word *resident* is used to describe a person who is being cared for in a long-term care setting because the long-term care facility becomes the person's home, either temporarily or permanently.
- The word *client* is used to describe a person who is being cared for in his or her home.

Structure of health care organizations

Most health care organizations are set up in a way similar to that shown in Figure 1-3. Most are governed by a board of trustees (also called a board of directors), and most have divisions (groups in charge of certain aspects of the organization's function). An administrator or chief executive officer (CEO) usually manages the organization and is the link between the board and the rest of the organization.

The board is made up of community members. It sets policies to ensure that the care offered by the organization is safe and of good quality. The board also makes sure that the organization meets the needs of the community.

TABLE 1-1	Types of Health Care Organizations	
	TYPE OF ORGANIZATION	**DESCRIPTION**
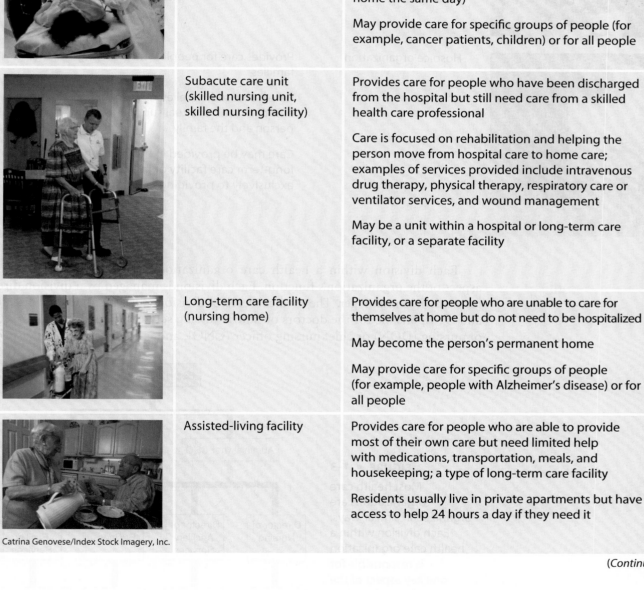	Hospital	Provides care for people with acute medical or surgical conditions Provides inpatient care (the person stays for one or more nights) or outpatient care (the person comes to the hospital for a scheduled treatment and then goes home the same day) May provide care for specific groups of people (for example, cancer patients, children) or for all people
	Subacute care unit (skilled nursing unit, skilled nursing facility)	Provides care for people who have been discharged from the hospital but still need care from a skilled health care professional Care is focused on rehabilitation and helping the person move from hospital care to home care; examples of services provided include intravenous drug therapy, physical therapy, respiratory care or ventilator services, and wound management May be a unit within a hospital or long-term care facility, or a separate facility
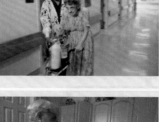	Long-term care facility (nursing home)	Provides care for people who are unable to care for themselves at home but do not need to be hospitalized May become the person's permanent home May provide care for specific groups of people (for example, people with Alzheimer's disease) or for all people
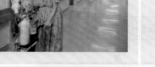	Assisted-living facility	Provides care for people who are able to provide most of their own care but need limited help with medications, transportation, meals, and housekeeping; a type of long-term care facility Residents usually live in private apartments but have access to help 24 hours a day if they need it

Catrina Genovese/Index Stock Imagery, Inc.

(Continued)

TABLE 1-1	**Types of Health Care Organizations** (*Continued*)	
	TYPE OF ORGANIZATION	**DESCRIPTION**
	Home health care agency	Provides skilled care in a person's home Provides services for people of all ages with any number of different medical needs
	Hospice organization	Provides care for people who are dying and their families Care is focused on relieving pain and providing emotional and spiritual support for both the dying person and the family Care may be provided in the home, hospital, or long-term care facility or in a facility devoted exclusively to providing care to the dying

Each division within a health care organization is responsible for one key aspect of the organization's function. Each division is managed by a division director or division manager. The medical services division is led by a medical director, and is responsible for the doctors on staff. Nursing services is headed by a director of nursing (DON) or chief nursing officer (CNO), and is responsible for all aspects

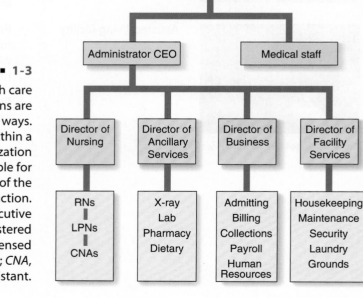

FIGURE ■ 1-3

Most health care organizations are organized in similar ways. Each division within a health care organization is responsible for one key aspect of the organization's function. *CEO*, chief executive officer; *RN*, registered nurse; *LPN*, licensed practical nurse; *CNA*, certified nursing assistant.

of the organization that have to do with patient or resident care. Business services is led by a business director, and usually oversees admissions, billing, and payroll. The business division may also oversee maintenance and housekeeping. The ancillary services division typically contains the departments in the organization that provide patient or resident services, such as social services and dietary services.

Putting it all together!

- Today, health care is delivered in the home through home health care agencies and hospice organizations. In addition, people can go to health care facilities such as hospitals, subacute care units, long-term care facilities ("nursing homes"), and assisted-living facilities to receive health care.

- Health care organizations are governed by a board of directors and have divisions that manage certain aspects of the organization's function.

PATIENTS, RESIDENTS, AND CLIENTS

What will you learn?

When you are finished with this section, you will be able to:

1. Discuss why people need health care.
2. Describe how the health care industry classifies people in need of its services.

Generally speaking, a person needing health care has some sort of illness, injury, or disability. These conditions can be either temporary or permanent. To make providing care more efficient, the health care industry groups people according to their age, illness or medical condition, or special health care needs:

- *Surgical patients* have illnesses or conditions, such as appendicitis or certain types of injuries, that are treated by surgery.
- *Medical patients* have an illness or a condition that is treated with methods other than surgery, such as medication, physical therapy, or radiation.
- *Obstetric patients* are those who are pregnant or have just given birth.
- *Pediatric patients* are children and adolescents.
- *Geriatric patients* are older adults, more than 65 years of age.
- *Psychiatric patients* are people with mental health disorders.
- *Rehabilitation patients* are those who are receiving therapy to restore their highest level of functioning.
- *Subacute* or *extended-care patients* do not need the total care provided by a hospital but are not quite ready to return home. They may need intravenous medications, physical therapy, or other treatments that cannot be provided by untrained caretakers.
- *Intensive care patients* are people who are critically ill and require highly skilled monitoring and care.

Putting it all together!

- Patients, residents, and clients are people who need the services of the health care industry because they are sick, injured, or unable to care for themselves.

- People in health care settings are grouped according to their age, illness or medical condition, or special health care needs.

OVERSIGHT OF THE HEALTH CARE SYSTEM

What will you learn?

When you are finished with this section you will be able to:

1. List some of the agencies that provide oversight of the health care system.

2. Describe how the survey process is used to monitor the quality of care given by health care organizations.

3. Discuss how government agencies help protect health care workers.

 4. Define the words United States Department of Health and Human Services (DHHS), Omnibus Budget Reconciliation Act (OBRA), the Joint Commission, Accreditation, Survey, and Occupational Safety and Health Administration (OSHA).

Today in the United States, many agencies exist to protect both the recipients and the providers of health care. Health care facilities must follow regulations set by the federal, state, and local governments. These regulations help to protect the entire community by making sure of the following:

- Providers of health care are properly trained and able to do their jobs.

- Health care facilities meet standards of cleanliness and quality.

- All products used in the delivery of health care are safe.

- Providers of health care are protected from on-the-job injuries.

- Quality health care is available to everyone.

The government monitors the activity of health care organizations and makes sure that organizations provide the type of care they say they provide. The government inspects health care organizations regularly to make sure that the standards are being followed. Any problems are addressed, and, if the problems are serious, the organization faces being fined or closed.

The **United States Department of Health and Human Services (DHHS)** is the primary government agency that is responsible for protecting this nation's health. The DHHS oversees many different agencies that are concerned with ensuring that quality health care is provided.

An in-depth investigation of long-term care facilities was carried out by the DHHS in response to complaints of neglect and abuse from people who had family members in long-term care facilities. This investigation resulted in a law known as the **Omnibus Budget Reconciliation Act (OBRA) of 1987**. OBRA improves the quality of life for people who live in long-term care facilities by making sure that residents receive a

United States Department of Health and Human Services (DHHS) ▪▪▪ the primary government agency responsible for protecting this nation's health; includes organizations such as the Food and Drug Administration (FDA), the Centers for Disease Control and Prevention (CDC), the National Institutes of Health (NIH), and the Centers for Medicare and Medicaid Services (CMS)

Omnibus Budget Reconciliation Act (OBRA) of 1987 ▪▪▪ an act passed in 1987 to improve the quality of life for people who live in long-term care facilities by making sure that residents receive a certain standard of care

certain standard of care. This care must take into account the residents' physical, emotional, spiritual, and social needs. OBRA also sets standards for the training and evaluation of nursing assistants who work in long-term care facilities. OBRA legislation is reviewed and passed by Congress each year. As you read this book, look for the OBRA icon, which highlights key information related to this law.

Several independent, nonprofit organizations also exist to help ensure that facilities provide quality health care. The largest and best-known of these independent organizations is **The Joint Commission** which sets national standards of all types of health care organizations and establishes expectations for how the organization carries out certain activities, especially activities that affect patient and resident safety and the quality of patient and resident care. Health care organizations request and pay for inspections by The Joint Commission. Those organizations that meet the standards receive **accreditation** by The Joint Commission and are permitted to display The Joint Commission's Gold Seal of Approval™, which is recognized nationwide as a symbol of quality (Fig. 1-4).

To ensure that a health care organization is meeting the established regulations, standards, or requirements set by the government agency or private organization that accredits or approves it, a survey process is utilized. A **survey** is an actual inspection and evaluation of a health care organization or facility. A *survey team* visits the facility and directly observes the care and services provided there. Afterward, a report is written up to show if there are any deficiencies that the facility must correct in order to maintain their accreditation status. If you work in an accredited health care facility, you will no doubt hear a lot about the survey process. In fact, many people will actually fear the survey process. However, if you are providing the type of quality care that you have been trained to do and are following the policies and procedures that have been established by your facility, you have nothing to be nervous about. Guidelines Box 1-1 lists ways that you can both excel in your job and help your facility do well during a survey regardless of the type of facility you work at.

The **Occupational Safety and Health Administration (OSHA)** is a government agency that is responsible for protecting the health and safety of American workers by enforcing standards and providing education to improve standards in the

The Joint Commission ■■■ an independent, nonprofit organization that sets national standards for all types of health care organizations and officially recognizes (accredits) organizations that meet these standards

Accreditation ■■■ official recognition that the organization meets certain standards of quality

Survey ■■■ an inspection of a nursing home carried out by the government to ensure that care is being provided according to standards and regulations

Occupational Safety and Health Administration (OSHA) ■■■ an agency within the Department of Labor that establishes safety and health standards for the workplace to protect the safety and health of employees

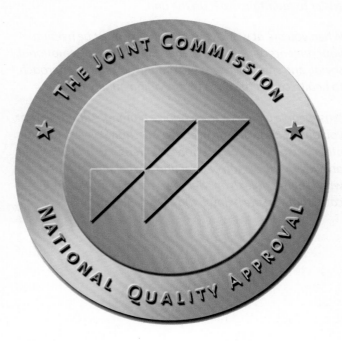

FIGURE ■ 1-4

Health care facilities that comply with the standards set by the Joint Commission are allowed to display the Joint Commission's Gold Seal of Approval.

Guidelines Box 1-1   Guidelines for Excelling at Your Job and Helping Your Facility Do Well During a Survey

What you do	Why you do it
Always act within your scope of practice, as defined by facility policy, your job description, and your state's regulations.	*This is the best way to ensure that the care you are providing is within the legal limits of your job.*
Always behave like the professional that you are. Be courteous and respectful toward others. Offer your assistance to patients or residents and coworkers readily. Have a positive attitude.	*Having a professional attitude and displaying a solid work ethic indicates to others that you take pride in your job and are interested in doing it to the best of your ability.*
Make sure that your conversations with coworkers are appropriate for the workplace. Be aware of the volume of your voice.	*You would not want anyone to overhear anything that would reflect poorly on you or your work ethic. Gossiping about others or going into great detail about your personal life is inappropriate in the workplace. Speaking in a loud voice adds to the noise level on the unit.*
When discussing a patient's or a resident's care with a coworker, be mindful of where the discussion is taking place and the volume of your voice.	*Discussions that involve a patient's or a resident's care need to be held in private areas to protect the resident's right to confidentiality.*
Do your part to maintain a neat and clean environment. Put items away after you use them. Dispose of trash properly. If you notice a spill or other mess, clean it up promptly.	*A cluttered, messy environment is unpleasant for everyone, patients or residents and staff alike. It may even present safety issues. It is difficult to work efficiently if you cannot locate something you need because it was not put away properly after the last person used it. If everyone on the unit does his or her part to keep the unit neat and clean, it is easier to maintain order on the unit.*
Always put your patient's or residents' needs first. Strive to provide humanistic, holistic care.	*When you are at work, your first priority must be helping your patients or residents to meet their physical, emotional, social, and spiritual needs. A humanistic, holistic approach to health care is the basis for providing quality care.*
Answer questions honestly and to the best of your ability. If you do not know the answer to a question, simply say that you do not know and offer your help in getting the person the answer he needs.	*Most people are quick to recognize bluffing. Admitting that you do not know the answer to a question conveys to the other person that you are honest. Offering to find out the answer for the person or directing the person to someone who is better able to answer the person's question indicates that you are helpful and conscientious.*

workplace. OSHA seeks to protect workers across all industries, not just the health care industry. You will see OSHA standards referenced frequently throughout this text. These standards protect you while you care for others.

Putting it all together!

- Government agencies set and enforce regulations and standards that help to protect both the people receiving health care and the people providing the care.
- The United States Department of Health and Human Services (DHHS) is the primary government agency responsible for protecting this nation's health and oversees many different aspects of health care.
- The Omnibus Budget Reconciliation Act (OBRA) ensures that people in long-term care facilities receive a certain standard of care.
- The Joint Commission sets national standards of all types of health care organizations and accredits those that meet these standards.
- The survey process is an actual on-site inspection of a health care organization by an accrediting organization.
- The Occupational Safety and Health Act helps to protect workers from on-the-job injuries.

PAYING FOR HEALTH CARE

What will you learn?

When you are finished with this section, you will be able to:

1. Discuss how health care is paid for.
2. Describe the difference between Medicare and Medicaid.
3. Explain how a Minimum Data Set (MDS) is used to justify Medicare reimbursement.

4. Define the words Medicare, Minimum Data Set (MDS), and Medicaid.

Health care can be expensive. Insurance can help to reduce these costs to the individual. As a nursing assistant, you should know how health care is paid for in the United States.

Private and group insurance

Although people can pay for health insurance privately using their own funds, many people participate in group insurance plans. *Group insurance* is insurance that is purchased at group rates by an employer or corporation. The employee may be covered in full as a benefit of employment or may pay for part of the coverage.

To reduce costs, many insurance companies use a *managed care system* to provide group insurance. Managed care systems help to deliver health care to people who need it by arranging contracts with various health care providers, who agree to provide services for a standard, reduced cost. Examples of managed care systems you might be familiar with include *preferred provider organizations (PPOs)* and *health maintenance organizations (HMOs)*.

Medicare

Medicare ■■■ a type of insurance plan that is federally funded by Social Security and which all people 65 years and older, and some younger disabled people, are eligible to participate in

Minimum Data Set (MDS) ■■■ a report that focuses on the degree of assistance or skilled care that each resident of a long-term care facility needs

Medicare is a type of insurance plan that is funded by the federal government. People who are 65 years or older are eligible for Medicare, regardless of their financial situation. Some younger people who are disabled also qualify for Medicare.

Health care facilities that are eligible to receive Medicare reimbursements must follow strict rules to receive payment. For example, to receive Medicare reimbursements, long-term care facilities must complete a **Minimum Data Set (MDS)** report for each resident in their care (Fig. 1-5). Information such as the person's weight, bowel and bladder habits, and ability to care for himself or herself is recorded regularly as part of the MDS report. Changes in these areas could indicate that a higher level of care is needed or that the person is not receiving the necessary care and, as a result, his or her condition is getting worse. One of your duties as a nursing assistant will be to accurately record the care that you give to patients and residents. Proper recording of the care you provide is necessary to ensure that the health care facility continues to receive Medicare reimbursements for the care provided.

Like insurance companies that insure the general public, the Medicare program is faced with the problem of controlling increasing health care costs. To help control these costs, Medicare has started a reimbursement program based on *diagnosis-related groups (DRGs)*. Under this system, payment for hospitalization, surgery, or other treatment is specified according to the diagnosis. Lengths of hospital stays are also determined by the diagnosis, and are typically short. Since being introduced by Medicare, the DRG system has been adopted by insurance companies in the private and group sectors as well, resulting in industry-wide changes. As a result of the DRG system, patients are discharged from the hospital sooner and sicker, a situation that has created an increased need for subacute care and home health care.

Medicaid

Medicaid ■■■ a federally funded and state-regulated plan designed to help people with low incomes to pay for health care

Medicaid is another type of insurance plan that is funded by the federal government. Medicaid helps people with low incomes to pay for health care. Elderly people, as well as those who are disabled, may also be eligible, especially if they have limited incomes. To receive Medicaid reimbursement, a facility must be approved by the state agency. Not all facilities or health care providers choose to participate in the Medicaid plan.

Putting it all together!

- Private and group insurance policies are one way that individuals pay for health care. Many group insurance policies rely on managed care systems, such as preferred provider organizations (PPOs) and health maintenance organizations (HMOs), to keep costs down.
- Medicare is a federally funded insurance plan for people who are 65 years of age and older and for some disabled people who are younger. Health care facilities must meet government regulations to receive Medicare reimbursement for services provided.
- Medicaid is a federally funded insurance plan for people with low incomes.

MINIMUM DATA SET (MDS) — *VERSION 2.0*
FOR NURSING HOME RESIDENT ASSESSMENT AND CARE SCREENING
FULL ASSESSMENT FORM
(Status in last 7 days, unless other time frame indicated)

SECTION A. IDENTIFICATION AND BACKGROUND INFORMATION

1.	RESIDENT NAME	a. (First) b. (Middle Initial) c. (Last) d. (Jr/Sr)
2.	ROOM NUMBER	
3.	ASSESS-MENT REFERENCE DATE	a. Last day of MDS observation period Month — Day — Year b. Original (0) or corrected copy of form (enter number of correction)
4a.	DATE OF REENTRY	Date of reentry from most recent temporary discharge to a hospital in last 90 days (or since last assessment or admission if less than 90 days) Month — Day — Year
5.	MARITAL STATUS	1. Never married 3. Widowed 5. Divorced 2. Married 4. Separated
6.	MEDICAL RECORD NO.	

7. CURRENT PAYMENT SOURCES FOR N.H. STAY (*Billing Office to indicate; check all that apply in last 30 days*)

Medicaid per diem	a.	VA per diem	f.	
Medicare per diem	b.	Self or family pays for full per diem	g.	
Medicare ancillary part A	c.	Medicaid resident liability or Medicare co-payment	h.	
Medicare ancillary part B	d.	Private insurance per diem (including co-payment)	i.	
CHAMPUS per diem	e.	Other per diem	j.	

8. REASONS FOR ASSESS-MENT
[*Note—If this is a discharge or reentry assessment, only a limited subset of MDS items need be completed*]

a. Primary reason for assessment
1. Admission assessment (required by day 14)
2. Annual assessment
3. Significant change in status assessment
4. Significant correction of prior full assessment
5. Quarterly review assessment
6. Discharged—return not anticipated
7. Discharged—return anticipated
8. Discharged prior to completing initial assessment
9. Reentry
10. Significant correction of prior quarterly assessment
0. *NONE OF ABOVE*

b. *Codes for assessments required for Medicare PPS or the State*
1. *Medicare 5 day assessment*
2. *Medicare 30 day assessment*
3. *Medicare 60 day assessment*
4. *Medicare 90 day assessment*
5. *Medicare readmission/return assessment*
6. *Other state required assessment*
7. *Medicare 14 day assessment*
8. *Other Medicare required assessment*

9. RESPONSI-BILITY/LEGAL GUARDIAN (*Check all that apply*)

Legal guardian	a.	Durable power attorney/financial	d.	
Other legal oversight	b.	Family member responsible	e.	
Durable power of attorney/health care	c.	Patient responsible for self	f.	
		NONE OF ABOVE	g.	

10. ADVANCED DIRECTIVES (*For those items with supporting **documentation** in the medical record, check all that apply*)

Living will	a.	Feeding restrictions	f.	
Do not resuscitate	b.	Medication restrictions	g.	
Do not hospitalize	c.	Other treatment restrictions	h.	
Organ donation	d.	*NONE OF ABOVE*	i.	
Autopsy request	e.			

SECTION B. COGNITIVE PATTERNS

1.	COMATOSE	(*Persistent vegetative state/no discernible consciousness*) 0. No 1. Yes (*If yes, skip to Section G*)
2.	MEMORY	(*Recall of what was learned or known*) a. Short-term memory OK—seems/appears to recall after 5 minutes 0. Memory OK 1. Memory problem b. Long-term memory OK—seems/appears to recall long past 0. Memory OK 1. Memory problem

3. MEMORY/RECALL ABILITY (*Check all that resident was **normally able to recall** during last 7 days*)

Current season	a.	That he/she is in a nursing home	d.
Location of own room	b.		
Staff names/faces	c.	*NONE OF ABOVE* are recalled	e.

4. COGNITIVE SKILLS FOR DAILY DECISION-MAKING (*Made decisions regarding tasks of daily life*)
0. *INDEPENDENT*—decisions consistent/reasonable
1. *MODIFIED INDEPENDENCE*—some difficulty in new situations only
2. *MODERATELY IMPAIRED*—decisions poor; cues/supervision required
3. *SEVERELY IMPAIRED*—never/rarely made decisions

5. INDICATORS OF DELIRIUM—PERIODIC DISOR-DERED THINKING/AWARENESS (*Code for behavior in the last 7 days*) [*Note: Accurate assessment requires conversations with staff and family who have direct knowledge of resident's behavior over this time*].
0. Behavior not present
1. Behavior present, not of recent onset
2. Behavior present, over last 7 days appears different from resident's usual functioning (e.g., new onset or worsening)

a. EASILY DISTRACTED—(e.g., difficulty paying attention; gets sidetracked)
b. PERIODS OF ALTERED PERCEPTION OR AWARENESS OF SURROUNDINGS—(e.g., moves lips or talks to someone not present; believes he/she is somewhere else; confuses night and day)
c. EPISODES OF DISORGANIZED SPEECH—(e.g., speech is incoherent, nonsensical, irrelevant, or rambling from subject to subject; loses train of thought)
d. PERIODS OF RESTLESSNESS—(e.g., fidgeting or picking at skin, clothing, napkins, etc; frequent position changes; repetitive physical movements or calling out)
e. PERIODS OF LETHARGY—(e.g., sluggishness; staring into space; difficult to arouse; little body movement)
f. MENTAL FUNCTION VARIES OVER THE COURSE OF THE DAY—(e.g., sometimes better, sometimes worse; behaviors sometimes present, sometimes not)

6. CHANGE IN COGNITIVE STATUS Resident's cognitive status, skills, or abilities have changed as compared to status of **90 days** ago (or since last assessment if less than 90 days)
0. No change 1. Improved 2. Deteriorated

SECTION C. COMMUNICATION/HEARING PATTERNS

1. HEARING (*With hearing appliance, if used*)
0. *HEARS ADEQUATELY*—normal talk, TV, phone
1. *MINIMAL DIFFICULTY* when not in quiet setting
2. *HEARS IN SPECIAL SITUATIONS ONLY*—speaker has to adjust tonal quality and speak distinctly
3. *HIGHLY IMPAIRED/*absence of useful hearing

2. COMMUNI-CATION DEVICES/TECH-NIQUES (*Check all that apply during last 7 days*)

Hearing aid, present and used	a.
Hearing aid, present and not used regularly	b.
Other receptive comm. techniques used (e.g., lip reading)	c.
NONE OF ABOVE	d.

3. MODES OF EXPRESSION (*Check all used by resident to make needs known*)

Speech	a.	Signs/gestures/sounds	d.
Writing messages to express or clarify needs	b.	Communication board	e.
American sign language or Braille	c.	Other	f.
		NONE OF ABOVE	g.

4. MAKING SELF UNDER-STOOD (*Expressing information content—however able*)
0. *UNDERSTOOD*
1. *USUALLY UNDERSTOOD*—difficulty finding words or finishing thoughts
2. *SOMETIMES UNDERSTOOD*—ability is limited to making concrete requests
3. *RARELY/NEVER UNDERSTOOD*

5. SPEECH CLARITY (*Code for speech in the last 7 days*)
0. *CLEAR SPEECH*—distinct, intelligible words
1. *UNCLEAR SPEECH*—slurred, mumbled words
2. *NO SPEECH*—absence of spoken words

6. ABILITY TO UNDER-STAND OTHERS (*Understanding verbal information content—however able*)
0. *UNDERSTANDS*
1. *USUALLY UNDERSTANDS*—may miss some part/intent of message
2. *SOMETIMES UNDERSTANDS*—responds adequately to simple, direct communication
3. *RARELY/NEVER UNDERSTANDS*

7. CHANGE IN COMMUNI-CATION/HEARING Resident's ability to express, understand, or hear information has changed as compared to status of **90 days** ago (or since last assessment if less than 90 days)
0. No change 1. Improved 2. Deteriorated

☐ = When box blank, must enter number or letter   a. = When letter in box, check if condition applies

MDS 2.0 September, 2000

FIGURE ■ 1-5 (*Continued on the next page*)

Nurses in long-term care facilities that receive Medicare funding must complete a Minimum Data Set (MDS) report for each resident in their care. This report is used to assess the amount of assistance that each resident needs. A nine-page form is used when the resident is first admitted to the facility. A shorter, three-page form is completed after 30, 60, and 90 days. The MDS report helps to make sure that the resident receives quality care that is directed toward his or her specific needs by requiring the nursing staff to evaluate those needs at regular intervals.

Resident _____   Numeric Identifier _____

SECTION D. VISION PATTERNS

1.	VISION	*(Ability to see in adequate light and with glasses if used)* 0. *ADEQUATE*—sees fine detail, including regular print in newspapers/books 1. *IMPAIRED*—sees large print, but not regular print in newspapers/books 2. *MODERATELY IMPAIRED*—limited vision; not able to see newspaper headlines, but can identify objects 3. *HIGHLY IMPAIRED*—object identification in question, but eyes appear to follow objects 4. *SEVERELY IMPAIRED*—no vision or sees only light, colors, or shapes; eyes do not appear to follow objects	
2.	VISUAL LIMITATIONS/ DIFFICULTIES	Side vision problems—decreased peripheral vision (e.g., leaves food on one side of tray, difficulty traveling, bumps into people and objects, misjudges placement of chair when seating self)	a.
		Experiences any of following: sees halos or rings around lights; sees flashes of light; sees "curtains" over eyes	b.
		NONE OF ABOVE	c.
3.	VISUAL APPLIANCES	Glasses; contact lenses; magnifying glass 0. No 1. Yes	

SECTION E. MOOD AND BEHAVIOR PATTERNS

1.	INDICATORS OF DEPRES-SION, ANXIETY, SAD MOOD	*(Code for indicators observed in last 30 days, irrespective of the assumed cause)* 0. Indicator not exhibited in last 30 days 1. Indicator of this type exhibited up to five days a week 2. Indicator of this type exhibited daily or almost daily (6, 7 days a week)			

VERBAL EXPRESSIONS OF DISTRESS		h. Repetitive health complaints—e.g., persistently seeks medical attention, obsessive concern with body functions	
a. Resident made negative statements—e.g., "*Nothing matters; Would rather be dead; What's the use; Regrets having lived so long; Let me die*"		i. Repetitive anxious complaints/concerns (non-health related) e.g., persistently seeks attention/reassurance regarding schedules, meals, laundry, clothing, relationship issues	
b. Repetitive questions—e.g., "*Where do I go; What do I do?*"		**SLEEP-CYCLE ISSUES**	
c. Repetitive verbalizations—e.g., calling out for help, ("*God help me*")		j. Unpleasant mood in morning	
d. Persistent anger with self or others—e.g., easily annoyed, anger at placement in nursing home; anger at care received		k. Insomnia/change in usual sleep pattern	
		SAD, APATHETIC, ANXIOUS APPEARANCE	
e. Self deprecation—e.g., "*I am nothing; I am of no use to anyone*"		l. Sad, pained, worried facial expressions—e.g., furrowed brows	
		m. Crying, tearfulness	
f. Expressions of what appear to be unrealistic fears—e.g., fear of being abandoned, left alone, being with others		n. Repetitive physical movements—e.g., pacing, hand wringing, restlessness, fidgeting, picking	
		LOSS OF INTEREST	
g. Recurrent statements that something terrible is about to happen—e.g., believes he or she is about to die, have a heart attack		o. Withdrawal from activities of interest—e.g., no interest in long standing activities or being with family/friends	
		p. Reduced social interaction	

2.	MOOD PERSIS-TENCE	One or more **indicators** of depressed, sad or anxious mood **were not easily altered by attempts to "cheer up", console, or reassure the resident over last 7 days** 0. No mood 1. Indicators present, 2. Indicators present, indicators not easily altered	
3.	CHANGE IN MOOD	Resident's mood status has changed as compared to status of 90 days ago (or since last assessment if less than 90 days) 0. No change 1. Improved 2. Deteriorated	
4.	BEHAVIORAL SYMPTOMS	(A) *Behavioral* symptom *frequency in last 7 days* 0. Behavior not exhibited in last 7 days 1. Behavior of this type occurred 1 to 3 days in last 7 days 2. Behavior of this type occurred 4 to 6 days, but less than daily 3. Behavior of this type occurred daily		

		(B) *Behavioral* symptom *alterability in last 7 days* 0. Behavior not present OR behavior was easily altered 1. Behavior was not easily altered	(A)	(B)
		a. WANDERING (moved with no rational purpose, seemingly oblivious to needs or safety)		
		b. VERBALLY ABUSIVE BEHAVIORAL SYMPTOMS (others were threatened, screamed at, cursed at)		
		c. PHYSICALLY ABUSIVE BEHAVIORAL SYMPTOMS (others were hit, shoved, scratched, sexually abused)		
		d. SOCIALLY INAPPROPRIATE/DISRUPTIVE BEHAVIORAL SYMPTOMS (made disruptive sounds, noisiness, screaming, self-abusive acts, sexual behavior or disrobing in public, smeared/threw food/feces, hoarding, rummaged through others' belongings)		
		e. RESISTS CARE (resisted taking medications/ injections, ADL assistance, or eating)		

5.	CHANGE IN BEHAVIORAL SYMPTOMS	Resident's behavior status has changed as compared to **status of 90 days ago** (or since last assessment if less than 90 days) 0. No change 1. Improved 2. Deteriorated	

SECTION F. PSYCHOSOCIAL WELL-BEING

1.	SENSE OF INITIATIVE/ INVOLVE-MENT	At ease interacting with others	a.
		At ease doing planned or structured activities	b.
		At ease doing self-initiated activities	c.
		Establishes own goals	d.
		Pursues involvement in life of facility (e.g., makes/keeps friends; involved in group activities; responds positively to new activities; assists at religious services)	e.
		Accepts invitations into most group activities	f.
		NONE OF ABOVE	g.
2.	UNSETTLED RELATION-SHIPS	Covert/open conflict with or repeated criticism of staff	a.
		Unhappy with roommate	b.
		Unhappy with residents other than roommate	c.
		Openly expresses conflict/anger with family/friends	d.
		Absence of personal contact with family/friends	e.
		Recent loss of close family member/friend	f.
		Does not adjust easily to change in routines	g.
			h.
3.	PAST ROLES	Strong identification with past roles and life status	a.
		Expresses sadness/anger/empty feeling over lost roles/status	b.
		Resident perceives that daily routine (customary routine, activities) is very different from prior pattern in the community	c.
		NONE OF ABOVE	d.

SECTION G. PHYSICAL FUNCTIONING AND STRUCTURAL PROBLEMS

1.	(A) ADL SELF-PERFORMANCE—(*Code for resident's PERFORMANCE OVER ALL SHIFTS during last 7 days—Not including setup*) 0. *INDEPENDENT*—No help or oversight —OR— Help/oversight provided only 1 or 2 times during last 7 days 1. *SUPERVISION*—Oversight, encouragement or cueing provided 3 or more times during last 7 days —OR— Supervision (3 or more times) plus physical assistance provided only 1 or 2 times during last 7 days 2. *LIMITED ASSISTANCE*—Resident highly involved in activity; received physical help in guided maneuvering of limbs or other nonweight bearing assistance 3 or more times — OR—More help provided only 1 or 2 times during last 7 days 3. *EXTENSIVE ASSISTANCE*—While resident performed part of activity, over last 7-day period, help of following type(s) provided 3 or more times: — Weight-bearing support — Full staff performance during part (but not all) of last 7 days 4. *TOTAL DEPENDENCE*—Full staff performance of activity during entire 7 days 8. *ACTIVITY DID NOT OCCUR* during entire 7 days

	(B) ADL SUPPORT PROVIDED—(*Code for MOST SUPPORT PROVIDED OVER ALL SHIFTS during last 7 days; code regardless of resident's self-performance classification*) 0. No setup or physical help from staff 1. Setup help only 2. One person physical assist 8. ADL activity itself did not 3. Two+ persons physical assist occur during entire 7 days	(A) SELF-PERF	(B) SUPPORT
a.	BED MOBILITY	How resident moves to and from lying position, turns side to side, and positions body while in bed		
b.	TRANSFER	How resident moves between surfaces—to/from: bed, chair, wheelchair, standing position (EXCLUDE to/from bath/toilet)		
c.	WALK IN ROOM	How resident walks between locations in his/her room		
d.	WALK IN CORRIDOR	How resident walks in corridor on unit		
e.	LOCOMO-TION ON UNIT	How resident moves between locations in his/her room and adjacent corridor on same floor. If in wheelchair, self-sufficiency once in chair		
f.	LOCOMO-TION OFF UNIT	How resident moves to and returns from off unit locations (e.g., areas set aside for dining, activities, or treatments). **If facility has only one floor, how resident moves to and from distant areas on the floor. If in wheelchair, self-sufficiency once in chair**		
g.	DRESSING	How resident puts on, fastens, and takes off all items of **street clothing**, including donning/removing prosthesis		
h.	EATING	How resident eats and drinks (regardless of skill). Includes intake of nourishment by other means (e.g., tube feeding, total parenteral nutrition)		
i.	TOILET USE	How resident uses the toilet room (or commode, bedpan, urinal); transfer on/off toilet, cleanses, changes pad, manages ostomy or catheter, adjusts clothes		
j.	PERSONAL HYGIENE	How resident maintains personal hygiene, including combing hair, brushing teeth, shaving, applying makeup, washing/drying face, hands, and perineum (EXCLUDE baths and showers)		

MDS 2.0 September, 2000

FIGURE ■ 1-5 *(Continued)*

What did you learn?

Multiple Choice

Select the single best answer for each of the following questions.

1. Who is the focus of the health care team's efforts?
   a. The doctor
   b. The director of nursing
   c. The organization's board of trustees
   d. The patient or resident

2. What does the Occupational Safety and Health Administration do?
   a. Sets standards for the education of nursing assistants
   b. Ensures that the rights of patients and residents are upheld
   c. Makes sure that organizations follow safety and health standards designed to keep workers safe
   d. Sets policies to ensure that the care offered by the organization is safe and of good quality

3. The inspection of a nursing home carried out by the government to insure that care is being provided according to standards and regulations is called a/an:
   a. OBRA requirement
   b. survey
   c. sentinel event
   d. MDS report

Matching

Match each type of health care facility with its description.

_____ 1. Assisted-living facility

_____ 2. Long-term care facility (nursing home)

_____ 3. Hospice organization

_____ 4. Home health care agency

_____ 5. Subacute care unit (skilled nursing unit, skilled nursing facility)

a. Place where people who can provide for most of their own care but who need limited assistance can live

b. Provides skilled care in a person's home

c. Provides care for people who cannot care for themselves but are not ill enough to be hospitalized

d. Provides care for people who are dying and their families

e. Provides care that is focused on rehabilitation; assists patients in making the transition from hospital care to home care

Match each vocabulary word with its definition.

_____ 1. Holistic

_____ 2. Minimum Data Set

_____ 3. Omnibus Budget Reconciliation Act

_____ 4. Medicare

_____ 5. Medicaid

a. Improves the quality of life for people who live in long-term care facilities by making sure that they receive a certain standard of care

b. A federally funded and state-regulated insurance plan designed to help people with low incomes pay for health care

c. Care of the whole person, physically and emotionally

d. A federally funded insurance plan in which all people 65 years or older and some younger disabled people are eligible to participate

e. A report that focuses on the degree of assistance or skilled care that each resident of a long-term care facility needs

 Stop **and** Think!

Think about what health care was like in the United States 100 years ago. How has health care delivery changed in the United States since the early 1900s? What aspects of the "old-fashioned" way of delivering health care were good? Not so good? What aspects of modern health care delivery are good? Not so good?

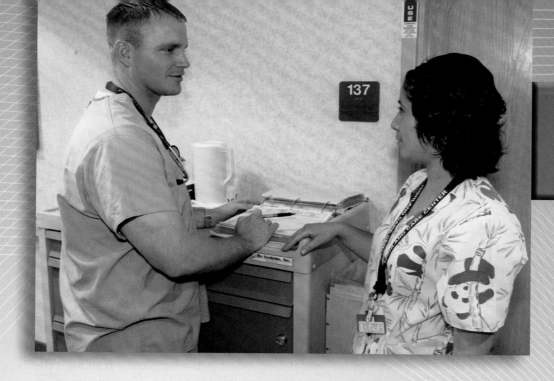

CHAPTER 2

Nurses and nursing assistants work together to provide safe, competent patient or resident care.

The Nursing Assistant's Job

As a nursing assistant, you will be responsible for providing safe, quality care to your patients or residents. In this chapter, you will learn about the education that is needed to work as a nursing assistant. You will also learn about how the nursing assistant works as a member of the nursing team, and about some of the legal and ethical aspects of the nursing assistant's job.

EDUCATION OF THE NURSING ASSISTANT

What will you learn?

When you are finished with this section, you will be able to:

1. Discuss the Omnibus Budget Reconciliation Act (OBRA) requirements for nursing assistant training.
2. Describe the certification process.
3. Describe the contents of the registry.
4. Define the words competency evaluation, reciprocity, and registry.

Training and certification

The Omnibus Budget Reconciliation Act (OBRA) requires all nursing assistants who want to be employed in long-term care facilities to complete a training program and to pass a test that evaluates their knowledge and skills. A minimum of 75 hours of training is required. This training must include classroom lectures and hands-on practice of skills, as well as supervised experience in an actual health care setting (Fig. 2-1). Topics that are included as part of the required training include:

- Basic nursing skills, such as how to measure vital signs
- Personal care skills, such as assisting with bathing and grooming
- Safety and emergency procedures
- Infection control procedures
- Communication skills
- Patient and resident rights

The training ends with a competency evaluation. During the written portion of the competency evaluation, you will have to answer approximately 75 multiple-choice questions. During the skills portion, you will be asked to perform selected nursing

Competency evaluation ▪▪▪ an exam consisting of a written portion and a skills portion that must be passed at the end of the nursing assistant training course to obtain certification

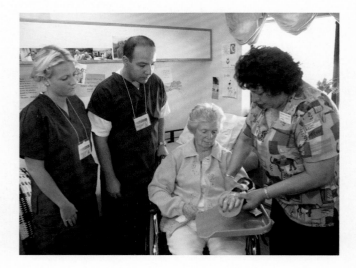

FIGURE ▪ 2-1

Part of a nursing assistant's training involves working with patients or residents in an actual health care setting.

skills. The actual number of test questions that you must answer and the skills that you must perform are determined by your state. OBRA specifies that you will have three chances to complete the evaluation successfully. The score that you must get to pass the evaluation varies from state to state.

In some cases, a person who has worked in a health care setting and already knows how to perform the duties required of a nursing assistant may be allowed to take the competency evaluation without completing the training program first. However, the person must pass both the written and the skills portions of the test on the first try. If he does not, then he must complete the course before taking the competency evaluation in again.

When you complete your training program and pass the competency evaluation, you will be certified to work as a nursing assistant in the state where you completed your training and passed your competency evaluation. In many cases, you will be able to work in other states as well, due to the principle of **reciprocity**. Some states accept the OBRA minimum of 75 hours of training, while others require more hours. If you want to work in a state that requires more hours of training than you have, additional training can be obtained.

Reciprocity ▪▪▪ the principle by which one state recognizes the validity of a license or certification granted by another state

If you stop working as a nursing assistant for 2 or more years and then decide that you want to return to the profession, you will need to retake your training course and pass the competency evaluation again before you will be allowed to work.

✓ Registry

OBRA requires every state to maintain a **registry** that contains the following information about each nursing assistant:

- Full name, including maiden name and any married names
- Last known home address
- Social Security number
- Date of birth
- Date the competency evaluation was passed
- Reported incidents of resident abuse or neglect, or theft of resident property

Registry ▪▪▪ an official record, maintained by the state, of the people who have successfully completed the nursing assistant training program

Registry information can be requested by any long-term care facility needing the information. Information about performance concerns, such as resident abuse, must remain in the registry for at least 5 years.

> *The knowledge, skills, and responsibilities of the nursing assistant have grown over the years. The very first nursing assistants usually did not have training in the health care field, which led to poor care in many cases. Today's nursing assistants, however, are well-trained members of the health care team with many important responsibilities.*

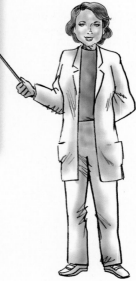

✓ Continuing education

Regular in-service education and performance reviews are also mandated by OBRA. Long-term care facilities must provide a minimum of 12 hours of in-service training per year to nursing assistants. During in-service training, new skills may be taught or existing skills reviewed, depending on the needs of the facility.

Putting it all together!

■ Educational standards, such as those set by OBRA, help to ensure that nursing assistants have the skills and knowledge they need to perform their jobs safely and competently.

THE NURSING ASSISTANT AS A MEMBER OF THE NURSING TEAM

What will you learn?

When you are finished with this section, you will be able to:

1. List the members of the nursing team, and describe the role of each team member.
2. Describe various ways that nursing teams work together in a health care setting.
3. List the steps of the nursing process, and describe how the nursing team uses the nursing process to plan the patient's or resident's care.
4. Discuss the delegation process as it relates to the nursing assistant.
5. List the five rights of delegation.

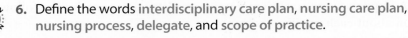

6. Define the words interdisciplinary care plan, nursing care plan, nursing process, delegate, and scope of practice.

How the nursing team works together

The nursing team, part of the health care team, is responsible for providing care to the patient or resident (Table 2-1). At a minimum, the nursing team consists of a nurse and a nursing assistant. The nursing assistant assists the nurse in giving care to patients or residents by performing basic nursing functions. The nurse may either be a *registered nurse (RN)* or a *licensed practical nurse (LPN)*. In some states, LPNs are called *licensed vocational nurses*, or *LVNs*. Other members of the nursing team may include a *charge nurse*, an RN or LPN/LVN who supervises the other nurses for a particular shift, and a *head nurse*, an RN who is in charge of a department or section. Each health care organization has an RN who directs all of the nursing care within that facility. This person is the *director of nursing (DON)*.

There are many different ways the members of the nursing team can work together:

■ In **primary nursing,** one nurse (an RN or LPN/LVN) is assigned several patients or residents and is responsible for planning and carrying out all aspects of care for those people. The nurse performs all of the nursing duties for his or her patients, from feeding and bathing to giving medications and other treatments. Other nurses and nursing assistants are responsible for the primary nurse's patients or residents when the primary nurse is not on duty, but all nursing efforts on behalf of those patients or residents are directed and coordinated by the primary nurse.

TABLE 2-1	The Nursing Team	
TEAM MEMBER	**REQUIREMENTS TO PRACTICE**	**CONTRIBUTION TO TEAM**
Registered nurse (RN)	A baccalaureate degree from a liberal arts college or university (4 years) OR An associate degree from a junior or community college (2 years) PLUS A license obtained by passing a state board examination	Develops nursing care plans and coordinates all aspects of patient or resident care Provides nursing care to patients or residents Delegates selected aspects of patient or resident care to other team members and supervises these team members as they carry out the delegated tasks
Licensed practical nurse (LPN) OR Licensed vocational nurse (LVN)	A certificate from a 12- to 18-month training program offered by a vocational school, community college, or hospital PLUS A license obtained by passing a state board examination	Under the supervision of a registered nurse (RN), provides nursing care to patients or residents Delegates selected aspects of patient or resident care to other team members and supervises these team members as they carry out the delegated tasks
Nursing assistant OR Patient care attendant Patient care technician (PCT) Nursing technician Nurse's aide Home health aide	A certificate from a 75- to 200-hour training program offered by a vocational school, community college, or health care facility, obtained by completing the training and passing a state-administered competency evaluation	Assists the RN or LPN with providing nursing care to patients or residents; responsibilities include basic nursing tasks related to meeting hygiene, safety, comfort, nutrition, exercise, and elimination needs

■ In **functional (modular) nursing,** each member of the nursing team carries out the same assigned task for all patients or residents. For example, for a particular group of patients or residents, one nurse may give all medications and another nurse may do assessments and special treatments. One nursing assistant may be assigned to take vital signs and assist with meals, while another nursing assistant may be assigned bathing and bedmaking tasks.

■ In **team nursing,** a team leader (an RN) determines all of the nursing needs for the patients or residents assigned to the team and assigns tasks according to each team member's skills and level of responsibility. For example, the nurse may assist the nursing assistant with bathing a patient or resident and then give that person his or her medication, or two nursing assistants may work together to complete the tasks usually handled by nursing assistants, such as bathing and bedmaking.

■ A recent trend being utilized in many health care facilities is known as "**patient-centered** or **patient-focused care.**" This method of nursing care is designed around the needs of the patient or resident and works to meet that person's needs more efficiently. Members of the nursing team are cross-trained to perform tasks that have in the past been done by other departments. For example, a nursing assistant may be trained to draw blood for laboratory tests or to do an EKG instead of relying on technicians from another department to come and perform those tasks.

Interdisciplinary care plan ▪▪▪ a specific plan of care for each patient or resident developed with input from all members of the health care team

Nursing care plan ▪▪▪ a specific plan of care for each patient or resident developed by the nursing team

Nursing process ▪▪▪ a process that allows members of the nursing team to communicate with each other regarding the patient's or resident's specific needs (in regard to nursing care), what steps will be taken to meet those needs, and whether or not the steps were effective in meeting the person's needs; it consists of five parts: assessment, diagnosis, planning, implementation, and evaluation

Delegate ▪▪▪ to authorize another person to perform a task on your behalf

The nursing process

The doctor is responsible for diagnosing a person's medical problems and ordering medication or other therapies to correct those problems. However, the actual coordination, planning, and implementation of that care require the efforts of other members of the health care team. Those members involved with the patient's or the resident's care may include nurses, nursing assistants, dietitians, social workers, and physical therapists. The patient or resident and his or her family members also play an important role in this process, especially in the long-term care setting. All health team members meet with the patient or the resident and family members to develop a specific, individualized plan of care called an interdisciplinary care plan. As part of the interdisciplinary care plan, the nursing team will then develop a specific plan of care for each patient or resident called the "nursing care plan."

The nursing process is used to create the nursing care plan. The five steps of the nursing process are described in Box 2-1. As a nursing assistant, you will be involved in the implementation step of the nursing process. You will also help the nurse with the assessment and evaluation steps of the nursing process by observing how your patients or residents are doing and reporting this information to the nurse.

Delegation

To ensure that the nursing team functions efficiently, an RN or LPN has the authority to delegate selected tasks to a nursing assistant. Typically, the nurse will delegate

---

Box 2-1   The Nursing Process

1. **Assessment.** During this step, the nurse gathers information about the patient or resident. As part of the assessment process, the nurse examines the patient or resident and asks questions about his or her abilities, level of discomfort, eating and toileting habits, and specific needs.

2. **Diagnosis.** Using the information gathered during the assessment step, the nurse then develops a *nursing diagnosis*, or a statement that describes a problem the person is having, as well as the cause of the problem. Unlike a medical diagnosis, which identifies a medical problem that must be managed by a doctor, a nursing diagnosis identifies a problem that the nursing staff can manage independently.

3. **Planning.** The next step in the nursing process involves making a plan for the person's care. Using information obtained from the nursing diagnosis, the nurse develops *interventions* (actions that will be taken to help the person) and *goals* (descriptions of what the interventions are meant to achieve). The interventions and goals that have been set for the patient or resident are written down in a formal way. This document is the nursing care plan.

4. **Implementation.** During the implementation step, the interventions that were detailed in the nursing care plan are carried out. (The nursing care plan specifies the team members who are responsible for doing each intervention.)

5. **Evaluation.** During the evaluation step, the nursing team checks the effectiveness of the nursing care plan and revises it as necessary. Is the care plan working? Are the goals being met? What needs to be improved or changed to meet the goals? Has the patient's or resident's status changed? Is the existing nursing care plan still appropriate for the patient or resident? If certain interventions are not working or if the goals have been met, the nursing care plan will change.

nursing tasks related to routine care (hygiene, comfort, exercise) to nursing assistants. An RN can also delegate certain nursing tasks, such as data collection and documentation, to a nursing assistant. However, nursing tasks that require professional judgment, such as assessment, planning, or evaluating, cannot be delegated to a nursing assistant. For example, a nursing assistant can take a person's vital signs and record this information on the person's chart, but the assistant is not qualified to interpret the data.

To help nurses make good decisions about which tasks to delegate and to whom, the National Council of State Boards of Nursing (NCSBN) has developed guidelines called the *five rights of delegation* (Table 2-2). You and the nurse share the responsibility for making sure that delegated tasks are carried out without causing harm to the patient or resident. The nurse is responsible for making good decisions about which tasks to delegate and for providing adequate supervision. You are responsible for recognizing which delegated tasks are within your **scope of practice** and range of abilities and using this knowledge as the basis for either accepting or refusing the assignment. Just as a nurse uses the five rights of delegation to decide which tasks to delegate and to whom, you can use the five rights of delegation to help you to decide whether to accept or decline a delegated task (see Table 2-2).

Scope of practice ■■■ the range of tasks that a nursing assistant is legally permitted to do

TABLE 2-2	Five Rights of Delegation	
	QUESTIONS THE NURSE MUST CONSIDER	**QUESTIONS THE NURSING ASSISTANT MUST CONSIDER**
The right task	Is this a task that can be delegated? Does the nurse's practice act in this state allow me to delegate the task? Is the task in the job description for the nursing assistant?	Does the state allow me to perform this task? Have I been trained to do this task? Do I have experience performing this task? Is this task in my job description?
The right circumstance	What is the patient's or resident's condition? Is he or she stable? What are the needs of the patient or resident at this time?	Can I perform this task safely, given the patient's or resident's condition?
The right person	Does the nursing assistant have the right training and experience to safely complete the task?	Am I confident that I can perform this task safely? Do I have any reservations about performing this task, and if so, what are they?
The right direction	Am I able to give the nursing assistant clear direction regarding how to perform this task? Am I able to explain to the nursing assistant what is expected?	Did the nurse give me clear instructions? Do I understand what the nurse expects?
The right supervision	Will I be available to supervise and answer questions?	Will the nurse be available to supervise and answer questions?

Box 2-2   Tasks that Are Generally Beyond the Nursing Assistant's Scope of Practice

Giving medications (including oxygen). Some states allow nursing assistants to give medications to residents in assisted-living facilities if the nursing assistant has received specialized training to do so. Generally, only a licensed nurse (RN or LPN) or doctor is allowed to give medications. Nursing assistants may assist patients in taking medication by bringing water or helping to open the medicine bottle.

Receiving verbal orders (in person or over the telephone) from doctors. Licensed nurses (RNs or LPNs) are the only personnel authorized to receive doctors' orders.

Diagnosing illness and prescribing treatments. Only doctors can diagnose illness and prescribe medical or surgical treatment.

Supervising other nursing assistants. Licensed nurses (RNs or LPNs) are responsible for supervising nursing assistants.

Performing procedures that require sterile technique. Nursing assistants are permitted to assist a nurse in performing a sterile procedure, but they are not trained to do these procedures themselves.

Inserting or removing tubes from a person's body (bladder, esophagus, trachea, nose, ears). Nursing assistants generally are not trained in procedures that involve inserting or removing tubes from a patient's or resident's body. Exceptions may be made if the nursing assistant has had the opportunity to practice a procedure under an instructor's supervision.

You should never refuse an assignment simply because you do not want to do it. You must have a good reason for refusing to carry out an assignment, or you could lose your job. Valid reasons for refusing an assignment include the following:

- The task is outside of your scope of practice. Box 2-2 summarizes tasks that are generally outside of the scope of practice of a nursing assistant.
- The task is illegal or unethical or could cause harm to the patient or resident.
- The nurse is not available to supervise your efforts.
- You do not have the proper equipment.
- The directions are not clear.
- You have not received adequate training about the task or the equipment used.

General guidelines for accepting or declining an assignment are given in Guidelines Box 2-1. A good general rule to keep in mind is that you should not perform any task that is not listed in your job description (Fig. 2-2). Make sure that you are familiar with your employer's policies and with your duties and obligations as listed in your job description. Be aware of the limits of practice for nursing assistants in your state. Ask your supervisor about anything you do not understand. Keeping yourself informed is critical to ensuring that the care you give is within the legal limits of your job and to protecting yourself as well as your patients or residents (Fig. 2-3).

If you must decline a task that you have been assigned to do, it is your responsibility to state clearly that you are not going to do the task and your reason why. Failure to communicate your refusal to complete a task to the person requesting your help can jeopardize the care or safety of the patient or resident. The person requesting your help assumes that you are doing the task, unless he or she hears otherwise. Declining a task is a discussion that you should have privately with the

Guidelines Box 2-1   Guidelines for Accepting or Declining an Assignment

What you do	Why you do it
Always ask the nurse for clarification if there is something you do not understand.	*It is your responsibility to make sure you know what is to be done and how it is to be done before going to the patient or resident.*
Never perform a task that you have not been taught to do, or that you feel uncomfortable doing, unless you are supervised by a nurse.	*The nurse is ultimately responsible for ensuring the patient's or resident's safety. This means that it is the nurse's responsibility to ensure that whoever is performing the task on his or her behalf is qualified to do so and capable. It is irresponsible for you to misrepresent your abilities or to proceed unsupervised with a task that you are not fully capable of doing well.*
Never ignore an assignment because you do not know how to perform the task or the task is beyond your scope of practice.	*The patient's or resident's needs must be attended to, either by you or by someone else. If you feel that you cannot perform the task that you are being asked to do, explain your concerns to the nurse so that he or she can either help you with the task or reassign it.*

person requesting the task of you. Do not discuss the issue in front of the resident, patient, or visitors.

When you agree to perform a task, you accept responsibility for your actions. If the task is within your scope of practice and you fail to perform the task properly, then you are responsible for any injury to the patient or resident that occurs. You must ask for help when you have questions or are unsure about how to proceed, and you must communicate with the nurse by reporting what you have done and what you observed.

Putting it all together!

- Nursing assistants are key members of the nursing team. Nursing assistants assist the nurse by performing basic functions, such as those related to hygiene, safety, comfort, nutrition, exercise, and elimination.
- The nursing team may organize their work according to the primary nursing model, the functional (modular) nursing model, the team nursing model, or use a patient-centered care approach.
- The nursing process is used by the nursing team to develop a plan of care for each patient or resident. The nursing process is ongoing, and the nursing care plan is adjusted as the patient's or resident's needs change. Nursing assistants participate in the nursing process by carrying out interventions and communicating information about the person's condition to the nurse.
- To ensure that the nursing team operates smoothly and efficiently, a "chain of command" exists. This means that licensed nurses (RNs or LPNs) are able to assign (delegate) certain tasks to nursing assistants.

(text continues on p. 31)

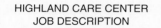

HIGHLAND CARE CENTER
JOB DESCRIPTION

CERTIFIED NURSING ASSISTANT (CNA)

SUPERVISOR : CHARGE NURSE/DIRECTOR OF NURSING

GENERAL QUALIFICATIONS

I. SKILL LEVEL AND EXPERIENCE:

A. Must be a Certified Nursing Assistant as required by state and federal law.
B. If applicant is an Aide in Training, certification must be obtained within 4 months of hire.
C. Must complete orientation required by company policy.
D. Must complete health screening and TB test (if required) within 2 weeks of employment.
E. Must complete a mandatory drug test within 90 days of hire.
F. Must be free of criminal activity proven by a criminal background check.
G. Must become familiar with and comply with all local, state, and federal regulations relating to the job.
H. Must obtain a current Food Handler's Permit within 14 days of hire.
I. Must show within 3 days of hire satisfactory evidence of identity and eligibility for employment.
J. Previous experience as a CNA and experience in working with geriatric residents is preferred and may be required.

II. COMMUNICATION AND DECISION-MAKING SKILLS:

A. Must possess the ability to work well and communicate effectively with other employees, residents, family members, visitors, government agencies, the general public, etc.
B. Must be able to read, write, speak, and understand English sufficiently to perform required duties.
C. Must be perceptive, with good judgment and decision-making/problem-solving skills.
D. Must be able to understand and implement the plan of care and assess resident needs.
E. Must be able to follow verbal and written instructions.

III. PERSONAL CHARACTERISTICS:

A. Must show courtesy and respect to other employees, residents, family members, visitors, government agencies, the general public, etc.
B. Must maintain good personal hygiene and dress and groom appropriately.
C. Must not be a habitual abuser of drugs (prescription or non-prescription) or alcohol.

IV. WORKING CONDITIONS & ENVIRONMENTAL PARAMETERS:

A. Must be very flexible and willing to cover shifts for other employees who are on vacation, sick, etc. Shift work will be required.
B. Must be willing to work holidays and weekends.
C. Must possess the ability to work in a wet or humid environment.
D. Must be able and willing to work with body fluids, excretions, extreme odors, etc., while using universal precautions.
E. Is subject to exposure to infectious waste, diseases, conditions, etc., including the AIDS and Hepatitis B viruses.
F. Must be able to relate to and work with the ill, disabled, elderly, emotionally upset, and, at times, hostile people within the facility.

V. PHYSICAL ABILITIES:

A. Must be able to sit, walk, run, lift and carry in excess of 75 pounds, bend, climb, kneel, squat, stoop, push, pull, grasp, reach arms above head, and have hand and finger dexterity.
B. Must be able to rapidly assist in the evacuation of all residents from the building in case of emergency.
C. Must be able to cope with the mental and emotional stress of working daily with geriatric residents and dealing with emergency situations.

FIGURE ▪ 2-2 *(Continued on the next page)*

Because a nursing assistant's duties can vary from state to state and also from facility to facility, it is always a good idea to be very familiar with your formal job description. Here is an example of a typical job description for a nursing assistant.

(Courtesy of Highland Care Center, Salt Lake City, Utah.)

D. Must be able to see, hear, and smell sufficiently to ensure the personal comfort, dignity, health, and safety of the residents, and to assure that the requirements of this position can be fully met.

E. Must be in good general heath and be emotionally stable.

F. Must be able to perform the essential job functions without posing a direct threat to residents, self, or others.

VI. EQUIPMENT TO BE USED:

Must be able to operate the following equipment: fire extinguisher, blood pressure cuff, stethoscope, weight chair, mechanical lift, thermometer, restraints, whirlpool bath, gait belt, hair dryer, rollers, curling iron, and other equipment as required to do the job.

> ### ESSENTIAL JOB FUNCTIONS

I. POLICIES:

A. Report on time as scheduled and follow all company policies and procedures.

B. Attend staff meetings and in-service sessions and complete 12 hours per year continuing education.

C. Become thoroughly familiar with emergency procedures and all applicable nursing procedures currently in use.

D. Must be able to perform duties in a timely fashion, and within the prescribed sequences and schedules.

E. Must be able to perform assigned tasks with a minimum of supervision and develop an awareness for and a willingness to perform other tasks, as needed, without constant supervision.

F. Must possess the ability to seek out new methods and principles and be willing to incorporate them into existing practices.

G. Must respect all resident rights, including the confidentiality of resident care information.

H. Follow all established safety precautions when operating equipment, and report hazardous and defective equipment or conditions to your supervisor.

I. Must be cooperative with other departments and be courteous and respectful in dealing with them at all times.

J. Report immediately to the Charge Nurse, to the Administrator, and to the proper legal authorities if you have reason to believe a resident has been physically, emotionally, or sexually abused, or been a victim of theft of their personal property.

K. Participate in and respond professionally to surveys (inspections) conducted by government agencies.

L. Create and maintain an atmosphere of warmth, cheerfulness, enthusiasm, and love, giving the resident the quality of service you would want to receive personally.

II. RESIDENT CARE:

A. The primary purpose of your position is to provide your assigned residents with routine daily nursing care in accordance with current regulations, established nursing care procedures, and as may be directed by your supervisors, and to provide quality resident care on a consistent basis.

B. Assume the authority, responsibility, and accountability necessary to carry out the assigned duties.

C. Assist residents as needed with activities of daily living. This includes bathing, hair care, nail care, oral care, shaving, dressing, eating, pericare, restraining (if ordered), assisting to and from bed, toileting, turning, transferring, lifting, changing when needed, etc.

D. Bathe each resident according to schedule. Change bed linens completely on bath days, more often as needed. Clean showers and tub rooms thoroughly before and after each use.

E. Make rounds regularly on each shift and assist each resident as needed, making sure they are safe, clean, and comfortable.

F. Always respect resident privacy and confidentiality including all details of resident care. Refer all questions regarding resident's status to the Charge Nurse and all questions regarding operation of care center to the Administrator.

G. Safeguard and use appropriately all resident belongings and appliances: hearing aids, eyeglasses, dentures, clothing, persona property, etc.

H. Escort residents to scheduled activities (recreational, religious, etc.) according to care plan.

I. Bring residents to the dining area, serve trays, feed residents as needed, and provide assistance to those not totally independent. Pick up trays and replace in kitchen cart for depository. Document meal intake percentage.

J. Fill resident water pitchers with ice water at least once a shift.

K. Perform restorative and rehabilitative nursing tasks as ordered. This includes turning and massaging bedfast residents every 2 hours, giving exercises as ordered, ambulating, checking and releasing restraints every 2 hours for 15 minutes, toileting every 2 hours or as ordered or as needed.

L. Inform the Charge Nurse of any observed change in resident's condition. This includes decrease in level of response, alteration in bowel function, skin lesions, changes in skin color or temperature, bruises, rashes, falls or other accidents, altered behavior, etc.

M. Accurately document all duties performed on the appropriate records. This includes flow sheets, charts, notes, accident reports, intake and output records, record of restraints, etc.

FIGURE ■ 2-2 *(Continued)*

III. LAUNDRY & CLEANING

   A. Make sure all resident clothing is properly marked and returned to the owner after being laundered.

   B. Take or send soiled linen and clothing to the laundry in properly secured laundry bags as soon as the bag is full and at the end of each shift, whether the bag is full or not. Linens soiled with feces, vomitus, blood, or any other bodily waste products must be thoroughly rinsed in the hopper room before being sent to the laundry.

   C. Keep resident rooms clean and orderly. (This includes nightstands, dressers, over-bed tables and closets.) Mop up spills and clean messes made by residents as needed.

   D. Help maintain cleanliness of work areas, break areas, and linen closets. Make sure that equipment and supplies are properly stored before leaving for breaks and at the end of each shift.

   E. If a resident has been discharged, have the cleaning staff completely clean and disinfect the area and get resident room ready for reoccupancy.

OTHER DUTIES

Perform other duties as may be assigned by the Charge Nurse or the Director of Nursing within the scope of CNA certification.

Check one

_____   I have read the above job description and can perform all duties as outlined.

_____   I have read the above job description and cannot perform the duties listed below and would like to discuss reasonable accommodation:

_____

_____

_____

| _____ | _____ |
| Signature | Date |

FIGURE ▪ 2-2 *(Continued)*

FIGURE ▪ 2-3

To stay within the legal limits of your job, know your scope of practice (as defined by the state and your job description), familiarize yourself with your employer's "policies and procedures" manual, and always seek clarification from your supervisor if there is something you do not understand.

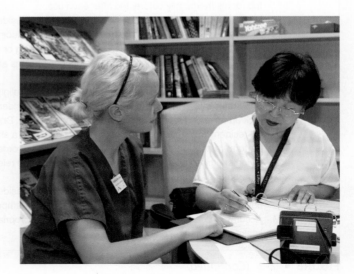

- The delegation of tasks cannot be taken lightly by either the nurse or the nursing assistant. Both share the responsibility for ensuring that the procedure is carried out without harm to the patient or resident.

- The nursing assistant must know which tasks are within his or her scope of practice and which tasks are not.

LEGAL AND ETHICAL ASPECTS OF THE NURSING ASSISTANT'S JOB

What will you learn?

When you are finished with this section, you will be able to:

1. List and discuss patients' rights as set forth in *A Patient's Bill of Rights*.

2. List and discuss residents' rights as set forth by the Omnibus Budget Reconciliation Act (OBRA).

3. Describe two major types of advance directives and explain why advance directives play an important role in health care.

4. Describe the seven violations of civil law that nursing assistants are at risk for committing in the workplace (defamation, assault, battery, fraud, false imprisonment, invasion of privacy, and larceny), and how to avoid each.

5. Define the types of abuse and describe signs that indicate abuse.

6. Discuss the health care worker's obligations in the reporting of suspected abuse.

7. Describe the ethical standards that govern the nursing profession.

8. Define the words decision-making capacity, advance directive, durable power of attorney for health care, living will, laws, civil laws, criminal laws, tort, unintentional tort, negligent, malpractice, intentional tort, slander, libel, informed consent, confidentiality, Health Insurance Portability and Accountability Act (HIPAA), abuse, ethics, and value.

Patients' and residents' rights

All of the people in our care have certain rights. In the hospital setting, these rights are listed in a document called *A Patient's Bill of Rights*, created by the American Hospital Association (AHA) in 1973 (Box 2-3). Since, 1973, the health care industry has changed dramatically, and "A Patient's Bill of Rights" has been revised to reflect those changes and is now called "The Patient Care Partnership". In a long-term care setting, these rights are included as part of the *Resident Rights* portion of OBRA (Box 2-4). Long-term care facilities that receive federal payments from Medicare must follow the *Resident Rights* portion of OBRA to be eligible to receive these payments. In respecting the rights of patients and residents, health care workers behave according to legal and ethical standards.

Box 2-3   A Patient's Bill of Rights

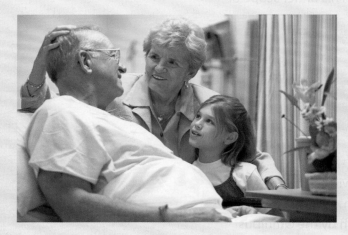

The patient has the right to:

1. Receive considerate and respectful care.
2. Have information about his diagnosis, treatment, and prognosis.
3. Make decisions about his plan of care and to refuse a recommended treatment.
4. Specify his wishes regarding his health care in advance in case the time comes when he can no longer make his wishes known himself.
5. Have privacy.
6. Expect that all communication (written and oral) related to his care will be treated with confidentiality.
7. Review the records related to his medical care and have the information they contain explained or interpreted as necessary.
8. Suggest alternatives to his planned care or transfer to another facility if he so desires.
9. Be informed of any business relationships between parties that influence the care he receives (for example, the hospital and an insurance provider).
10. Participate in, or decline to participate in, experimental studies.
11. Be informed of his options for care when he is discharged from the hospital.
12. Know how the hospital settles disputes, what the hospital charges for its services, and what options for payment are available.

In addition to having rights, the patient has responsibilities. The patient is responsible for:

1. Cooperating with health care providers.
2. Respecting the property, comfort, environment, and privacy of other patients.
3. Making an effort to understand and follow instructions concerning treatment.
4. Providing accurate and complete information about his health status by answering questions as truthfully and completely as possible.
5. Ensuring payment for services received (including providing insurance information in a cooperative and timely manner).
6. Informing the health care staff of any medications brought from home.
7. Accepting responsibility for the consequences of refused treatment or disregarded instructions.

Box 2-4   Resident Rights

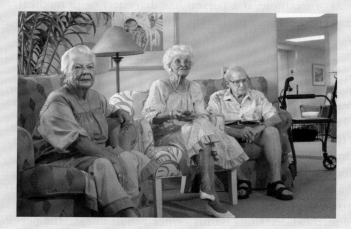

The resident has the right to:

1. Make decisions regarding her care, including choosing her doctor, participating in planning and implementing her care, having her individual needs and preferences accommodated, and voicing grievances about care.

2. Have privacy, including privacy while receiving treatments and nursing care, making and receiving telephone calls, sending and receiving mail, and receiving visitors; and to have personal and medical records treated confidentially.

3. Be free from physical or psychological abuse, including the improper use of restraints.

4. Receive visitors, and to share a room with a spouse if both partners are residents in the same facility.

5. Use personal possessions.

6. Control her finances.

7. Have information about eligibility for Medicare or Medicaid funds, and to be protected against Medicaid discrimination.

8. Have information about the facility's compliance with regulations, planned changes in living arrangements, and available services (and the fees for these services).

9. Remain in the facility unless transfer or discharge is required by a change in the resident's health, an inability of the resident to pay for the services she is receiving, or the facility is closed.

10. Organize and participate in groups organized by other residents or the families of residents and to participate in social, religious, and community activities of her choosing.

11. Have information about advocacy groups.

12. Choose to work at the facility, either as a volunteer or a paid employee (however, under no circumstances is a resident obligated to work in exchange for services).

Advance directives

Many patients and residents in health care facilities are not able to make their preferences for health care known, or they will become unable to make their preferences known in the future. For example, if a person has dementia or (a medical condition that results in the permanent and progressive loss of the ability to think and remember) experiences a loss of consciousness, the person will lose his or her decision-making capacity.

For these situations, state laws allow a person to make his or her wishes known through an advance directive. Examples of advance directives include a living will and durable power of attorney for health care.

A patient or resident may wish to give instructions about the type of care he or she wishes to receive in an effort to save his or her life, which may mean choosing to avoid "heroic measures" that will prolong life. The living will allows the person to ask that no life-sustaining treatments—such as cardiopulmonary resuscitation (CPR), mechanical ventilation, feeding tubes, or intravenous (IV) lines—be used to prolong his or her life.

A durable power of attorney for health care allows the patient or resident to name someone else to make medical decisions on his or her behalf in case the person is no longer able to make these decisions on his or her own. The designated person can be a family member, friend, or other trusted individual and may be called the person's *health care agent*.

Advance directives play a very important role in the health care setting, because many patients and residents have conditions that may result in either the temporary or permanent loss of their decision-making capacity. The *Patient Self-Determination Act of 1990* requires health care facilities to educate patients and residents about advance directives and to offer them the opportunity to establish a living will, a durable power of attorney for health care, or both.

Laws

One way the government works to protect its citizens' basic human rights is by making and enforcing laws. There are two types of laws: civil laws and criminal laws. People found guilty of violating civil laws usually must pay a fine or make a financial settlement to the party that was wronged. Those who violate criminal laws are often sentenced to prison.

Violations of civil law

When a patient or resident is admitted to a health care facility, he or she signs a form giving the facility permission to provide medical care. A health care worker employed by that facility likewise agrees to provide that care to the patient or resident. This arrangement is a contractual agreement. Contracts, such as the contract that exists between a nursing assistant and the person she or he cares for, are covered by civil law. When this civil law is violated, a *tort*, or wrong, is committed.

An unintentional tort occurs when someone causes harm or injury to another person or that person's property by accident. A person who commits an unintentional tort is considered negligent. For example, in each of the following scenarios, the nursing assistant would be considered negligent:

- A nursing assistant becomes distracted by another resident's needs and forgets to lock the wheels on the wheelchair she has just placed by the resident's bed. As the resident moves from the bed to the wheelchair, the wheelchair rolls, causing the resident to fall (Fig. 2-4).

Decision-making capacity ▪▪▪ the ability to make a thoughtful decision based on an understanding of the potential risks and benefits of taking a certain course of action

Advance directive ▪▪▪ a document that allows a person to make his or her wishes regarding health care known to family members and health care workers, in case the time comes when the person is no longer able to make those wishes known himself or herself

Living will ▪▪▪ a type of advance directive that states a person's wish that death not be artificially postponed

Durable power of attorney for health care ▪▪▪ a type of advance directive that transfers the responsibility for handling a person's affairs and making medical decisions to a family member, friend, or other trusted individual, in the event that the person is no longer able to make these decisions on his or her own behalf

Laws ▪▪▪ rules that are made by a governing authority, such as the state or federal government, with the intent of preserving basic human rights

Civil laws ▪▪▪ laws concerned with relationships between individuals

Criminal laws ▪▪▪ laws concerned with the relationship between the individual and society

Unintentional tort ▪▪▪ a violation of civil law that occurs when someone causes harm or injury to another person or that person's property without the intent to cause harm

Negligent ▪▪▪ word used to describe a person who fails to do what a "careful and reasonable" person would do in any given situation

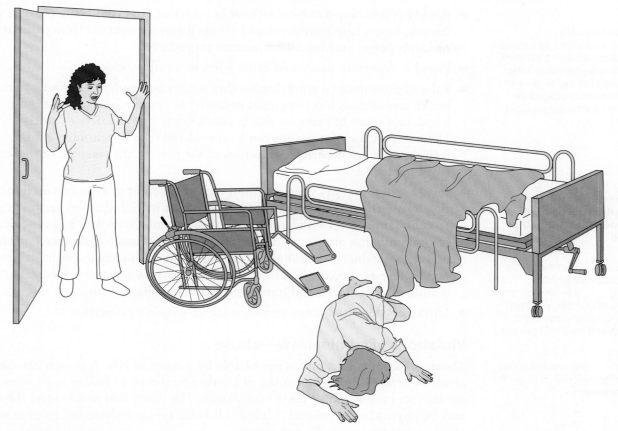

FIGURE ▪ 2-4

The nursing assistant who was responsible for this resident has committed an unintentional tort and would be considered negligent for failing to lock the wheels on the wheelchair, an action that would have prevented the resident from falling.

- While changing a resident's bed, a new nursing assistant forgets to check the linens for personal objects. As a result, the resident's dentures are sent to the laundry with the soiled linens, and the dentures are damaged when they go through the washing machine.

- A nursing assistant who is caring for a resident with a reputation for complaining fails to report the resident's complaints of pain to the nurse. It turns out that this time the resident's complaints were valid.

Negligence committed by people who hold licenses to practice their profession, such as doctors, nurses, lawyers, dentists, and pharmacists, is considered **malpractice**. Nursing assistants (who receive certification, but not licensure) are not charged with malpractice.

A violation of civil law committed by a person with the intent to do harm is considered an **intentional tort**. Intentional torts that nursing assistants are particularly at risk for committing in the workplace include the following:

- **Defamation** is making untrue statements that hurt another person's reputation. Defamation may take the form of **slander** or **libel**.

- **Assault** is threatening or attempting to touch a person without his or her consent, causing that person to fear bodily harm.

Malpractice ▪▪▪ negligence committed by people who hold licenses to practice their profession, such as doctors, nurses, lawyers, dentists, and pharmacists

Intentional tort ▪▪▪ a violation of civil law committed by a person with the intent to do harm

Slander ▪▪▪ spoken statements that injure someone's reputation; a form of defamation

Libel ▪▪▪ written statements that injure someone's reputation; a form of defamation

Informed consent ▪▪▪ permission granted by a patient or resident to begin treatment or perform a procedure after receiving a full explanation of the treatment or procedure from the health care provider

Confidentiality ▪▪▪ keeping personal information that someone shares with you to yourself

Health Insurance Portability and Accountability Act (HIPAA) ▪▪▪ a federal privacy regulation that helps to keep personal information about patients and residents private

Abuse ▪▪▪ the repetitive and deliberate infliction of injury on another person

- **Battery** is touching a person without her consent. To avoid being charged with battery, health care providers must obtain informed consent from patients and residents before starting a treatment or procedure.

- **Fraud** is deception that could cause harm to another person.

- **False imprisonment** is confining another person against his or her will. In the health care setting, it is sometimes necessary to confine a person to a chair, a bed, or a room to maintain that person's safety (or the safety of others). However, the use of restraints can be considered false imprisonment if the restraints are not needed for the safety of the patient, the resident, or the staff (see Chapter 12).

- **Invasion of privacy** is violating another person's right to keep certain information away from the examination of others (that is, violating the person's right to confidentiality). Confidentiality applies not only to spoken and observed information, but also to written information. The Health Insurance Portability and Accountability Act (HIPAA) of 1996 regulates who has the right to view a person's medical records and sets standards for how a person's medical information is to be stored and transmitted from one place to another.

- **Larceny** is theft (the act of stealing another person's property).

Violations of criminal law—abuse

Abuse is a criminal act and is punishable by a court of law. A person can commit abuse by *actively doing something* to another person or by *failing to do something for* another person. Abuse takes many forms. The injury that results from the abuse may be physical or emotional. Table 2-3 lists the types of abuse and gives examples of signs that abuse may be occurring.

RISK FACTORS FOR BECOMING A VICTIM OF ABUSE Anyone can become the victim of abuse, but those who depend on others for their care (the very young, the disabled, and the elderly) are particularly at risk. *Elder abuse* is the physical, emotional, or sexual abuse of an older person. *Child abuse* is the physical, emotional, or sexual abuse of a child. The more dependent the person is on others for care, the more at risk the person is for abuse or neglect.

RISK FACTORS FOR BECOMING ABUSIVE There are many reasons why a person may become abusive toward another. Sometimes, abuse is rooted in the desire of one person to overpower and dominate another. Many abusers were victims of abuse themselves. Other times, in a situation in which a person requires a great deal of care, the caregiver may become tired, frustrated, and overwhelmed by the responsibility of providing care, leading to abuse and neglect. This is often the case with an adult child who has to care for an ill and demanding elderly parent, without the proper training or support system.

Even people who are trained to give care may become overwhelmed by their responsibilities or a by particular situation. A health care worker is particularly at risk for becoming abusive when the patient or resident is "difficult" or hard to manage and the relationship is long term rather than short term. Regardless of the reason abuse occurs, abuse is never an acceptable form of behavior! Be very careful not to place yourself in the position of potentially abusing a patient or resident. Being found guilty of abuse could destroy your potential for future employment in the health care field.

ROLE OF THE NURSING ASSISTANT IN REPORTING ABUSE As a nursing assistant, you may find yourself in a situation in which you suspect that one of your patients or residents is being abused (Table 2-3). When this is the case, you are required by law to report your suspicions to the proper person in your facility. This person may be your supervisor or someone else. Follow your facility's policy. It is not your

TABLE 2-3	Types of Abuse	
TYPE OF ABUSE	**EXAMPLES**	**SIGNS THAT ABUSE MAY BE OCCURRING**
Physical abuse: Causing pain or injury to the person's body through the use of force	■ Hitting and slapping ■ Pushing and shoving ■ Pinching and kicking ■ Shaking ■ Burning ■ Force feeding ■ The inappropriate use of medications ■ The inappropriate use of physical restraints	■ Red marks, welts, or bruises, particularly on the face or torso ■ Broken bones ■ Broken or bent eyeglasses ■ Patches of missing hair ■ Laboratory work that indicates under- or overdosing of medications ■ Person displays fearful or anxious behavior, especially in the presence of the abuser ■ Person reports physical abuse
Neglect: Failing or refusing to provide for the person's basic human needs	■ Failing to provide food, water, clothing, shelter, or ordered medications ■ Failing to help the person meet hygiene and toileting needs ■ Withdrawing support or help from another person, in spite of duty or responsibility (abandonment)	■ Unusual weight loss ■ Dehydration ■ Pressure ulcers ■ Poor personal hygiene; unkempt appearance ■ Incontinence, dried feces on the skin, or skin irritation ■ Inadequate or inappropriate clothing for environment ■ Pain ■ Contractures ■ Uncontrolled medical conditions (possibly the result of a lack of prescribed medication or treatment) ■ Person reports improper care
Psychological (emotional) abuse: Causing emotional pain or injury through the use of words or actions	■ Insulting or threatening a person ■ Bullying, humiliating, or harassing a person ■ Treating a person in an undignified or childlike way ■ Giving a person the silent treatment ■ Isolating the person from others (involuntary seclusion)	■ Person appears emotionally upset (for example, the person cries frequently) ■ Person appears withdrawn or apathetic (does not seem to care about anything), or person stops responding ■ Changes in the person's behavior, or unusual behavior (such as rocking or biting) ■ Person reports psychological abuse

(Continued)

TABLE 2-3	Types of Abuse (*Continued*)	
TYPE OF ABUSE	**EXAMPLES**	**SIGNS THAT ABUSE MAY BE OCCURRING**
Sexual abuse: Subjecting the person to unwanted attention of a sexual nature, forcing the person to engage in unwanted sexual activity, or sexually exploiting the person (for example, by taking nude photographs of the person)	■ Touching personal body parts in an inappropriate way ■ Making inappropriate, sexually suggestive comments or gestures ■ Committing sexual assault or battery (for example, forced nudity, inappropriate photography, rape)	■ Bruising on breasts or in genital area ■ Torn or stained underwear ■ Unexplained bleeding from the vagina or rectum ■ Person reports sexual abuse or harassment
Financial abuse: Misusing or stealing another person's money or property	■ Stealing money or belongings ■ Withholding a person's Social Security checks or other sources of income ■ Making withdrawals from a person's bank account or cashing checks without the person's permission ■ Forging the person's signature on checks or legal documents ■ Tricking or blackmailing a person into giving away money or property ■ Tricking or blackmailing a person into signing a legal document or making changes to an existing legal document	■ Unexplained disappearance of money or belongings ■ Sudden change in bank account activity, such as unauthorized withdrawals from the person's account ■ Unexplained money or property transfers, or changes to the person's will ■ The inclusion of additional names on theperson's bank account ■ The discovery of forged documents ■ Person reports mishandling or loss of money or property

responsibility to investigate whether or not abuse has actually occurred or who has caused it. Your responsibility is to simply report your suspicions to the proper person.

Ethics

Ethics ■■■ moral principles or standards that govern conduct

Like laws, **ethics** guide our behavior in the workplace. The word "ethics" is derived from the Greek word *ethos*, which means "beliefs that guide life." Ethics helps us to determine the difference between right and wrong when there is no clear law or policy to tell us what to do. Each profession has a code of ethics. The code of ethics for nursing assistants is given in Box 2-5.

In addition, each person has a code of ethics that is derived from that person's **values**. Factors that influence a person's values include his or her religious or spiritual beliefs, level and type of education, culture and heritage, and life experiences.

Value ■■■ a cherished belief or principle

Box 2-5   Code of Ethics for Nursing Assistants

- Treat patients and residents with respect for their individual needs and values.

- Respect the patient's or resident's right to choice in regard to the individual's right to control his or her own care.

- Hold confidential all information about patients and residents learned in the health care setting.

- Be guided by consideration for the dignity of patients and residents.

- Fulfill the obligation to provide competent care to patients and residents.

As a nursing assistant, you need to think about how you feel about certain moral and ethical issues. Only then will you be able to understand that although another person's values may differ from yours, that person's values are as important to him or her as yours are to you. Ethical dilemmas can arise when we attempt to judge other people by our own ethical standards.

Putting it all together!

- Both the AHA's *Patient's Bill of Rights* and the *Resident Rights* portion of OBRA protect the people who receive our care. Health care workers are legally and ethically responsible for respecting the rights of patients and residents.

- Advance directives help to ensure that a person's wishes regarding end-of-life care are honored, even if the person is no longer able to express those wishes verbally.

- A living will states that the person does not want the health care team to take extreme measures to prolong his or her life.

- A durable power of attorney for health care allows the person to designate someone else to make medical decisions on his or her behalf.

- Laws and ethics guide our behavior in the workplace. Laws are rules established by a governing authority. Failing to obey these rules can result in punishment. Ethics refers to moral principles or standards that govern conduct. When we act according to ethical standards, we act in a certain way because we believe it is the right way to act, not because we risk punishment if we do not behave in that way.

- Civil laws are concerned with relationships between individuals. Violations of civil law are called torts. Torts may be intentional or unintentional.

- An unintentional tort occurs when someone causes harm or injury to another person or that person's property without the intent to do harm. A nursing assistant who commits an unintentional tort is considered negligent for failing to do what a careful and reasonable person would do.

- An intentional tort occurs when someone causes harm or injury to another person with the intent to do harm. Intentional torts that nursing assistants are particularly at risk for committing in the workplace include defamation, assault, battery, fraud, false imprisonment, invasion of privacy, and larceny.

- Abuse is a violation of criminal law. A nursing assistant who abuses a patient or resident could lose his or her job, as well as the potential for future employment in the health care field.

- Abuse can be physical, emotional, or sexual. Anyone can be a victim of abuse, but people who depend on others for their care (such as children, elderly people, and people with disabilities) are at high risk for abuse.

- Laws require any health care worker who suspects the abuse of a child or elderly person to report his or her suspicions to the proper authorities.

What did you learn?

Multiple Choice

Select the single best answer for each of the following questions.

1. Nursing assistants who work in the long-term care setting must complete a course of training and undergo a competency evaluation. These requirements are set by the:
   a. Centers for Disease Control and Prevention (CDC)
   b. Food and Drug Administration (FDA)
   c. Omnibus Budget Reconciliation Act (OBRA)
   d. Occupational Safety and Health Administration (OSHA)

2. As a nursing assistant, it is your responsibility to:
   a. Plan the patient's or resident's care
   b. Perform the tasks your supervisor assigns to you
   c. Do the best you can without asking for help
   d. Compare assignments with your co-workers

3. If you do not know how to do an assigned task, you should:
   a. Call another nursing assistant for help
   b. Ask the patient or resident how he or she prefers to have it done
   c. Decline to do the task
   d. Follow the instructions in the procedure manual

4. Nursing assistants work under the supervision of:
   a. A doctor
   b. A registered nurse (RN) or licensed practical nurse (LPN)
   c. Other nursing assistants
   d. The long-term care facility administrator

5. Which step of the nursing process involves gathering information about a patient or a resident?
   a. Implementation
   b. Assessment
   c. Planning
   d. Evaluation

6. To "delegate" means to:
   a. Do what you are told to do
   b. Give another person permission to perform a task on your behalf
   c. Transfer your duties to another assistant
   d. Have the charge nurse take your assignment

7. What information is included in the registry?
   a. The nursing assistant's full name
   b. The nursing assistant's Social Security number
   c. Any reported incidents of abuse or theft
   d. All of the above

8. All of the following are legal terms that relate to making false statements that injure another person's reputation except:
   a. Defamation
   b. Assault
   c. Slander
   d. Libel

9. If a registered nurse (RN) fails to raise the side rails on the bed of a confused patient and the patient falls out of bed and is injured, the nurse may be charged with:
   a. Malpractice
   b. Negligence
   c. An intentional tort
   d. Assault

10. *Resident Rights* are a part of which legislation?
    a. American Medical Association (AMA)
    b. Omnibus Budget Reconciliation Act (OBRA)
    c. Federal Emergency Management Agency (FEMA)
    d. Social Security Act

11. Which of the following is a basic right of residents?
    a. Right to choice
    b. Right to privacy and confidentiality
    c. Right to be free from verbal abuse, or any other abuse
    d. All of the above

12. Confidentiality means:
    a. Only sharing information with those directly involved in a patient's or resident's care
    b. Respecting a patient's or resident's right to privacy
    c. Never sharing information with anyone
    d. Both a and b

13. You are a nursing assistant working in a home health care setting. You suspect that one of your clients is being emotionally and physically abused by her husband. What should you do first?
    a. Call the police
    b. Keep your suspicions to yourself but continue to observe the situation
    c. Immediately report your suspicions to the case manager
    d. Tell another nursing assistant at the agency

14. One of your co-workers has been having a very hard time with one of her residents. The resident is confused and, as a result, is being uncooperative. In a moment of complete frustration, your co-worker says to the resident, "If you don't shut up and behave yourself right now, I'm going to slap you!" What kind of an intentional tort has this nursing assistant committed?
    a. Assault
    b. Battery
    c. Negligence
    d. Malpractice

15. A nursing assistant answers the telephone at the nursing station. The doctor who is calling wants to give a verbal order, and the nursing assistant tells the doctor that she is a nurse and can take the order. What intentional tort has the nursing assistant committed?
    a. Slander
    b. Fraud
    c. Libel
    d. Informed consent

16. What does the Health Insurance Portability and Accountability Act (HIPAA) protect?
    a. The patient's or resident's right to privacy
    b. The patient's or resident's right to sue negligent health care workers
    c. The patient's or resident's right to be free from abuse
    d. The patient's or resident's right to choose who will provide his or her care

17. A legal document that transfers the responsibility for handling a person's medical decisions to a family member, friend, or other trusted individual is known as a:
    a. Living will
    b. HIPAA agreement
    c. Form of consent
    d. Durable power of attorney for health care

 Stop **and** Think!

A licensed practical nurse (LPN) who works with you in a long-term care facility stops in Mrs. Taylor's room to give Mrs. Taylor her daily medications. Mrs. Taylor is in the bathroom and you are changing the linens on her bed. The nurse hands you the medication cup, which contains three pills, and asks you to have Mrs. Taylor take the pills as soon as she comes out of the bathroom. You are aware that in your state, nursing assistants who work in long-term care facilities are not allowed to give medications. When you mention your concern about giving Mrs. Taylor her medication to the nurse, she says, "It's okay; the other nursing assistants do this for me all of the time." What should you do?

 Stop **and** Think!

You have just received your assignment for the shift. Another assistant does not like her assignment and asks to switch residents with you. This makes you uncomfortable because you have just started at the facility and do not know if switching assignments is permitted. What should you do?

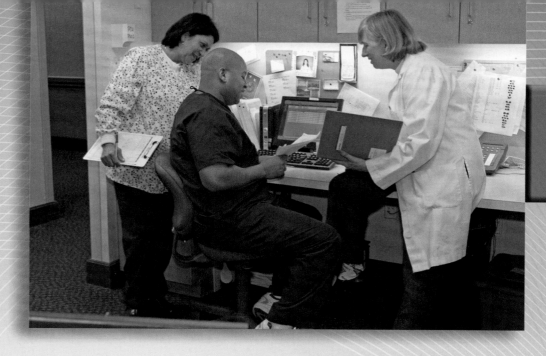

CHAPTER 3

The health care industry relies on all types of professionals to provide quality care to patients and residents.

Professionalism and Job-Seeking Skills

The health care field relies on all types of professionals, including nursing assistants, to provide quality care to patients and residents. In this chapter, you will learn about what it means to be a "professional" and what personal qualities you will need to succeed in the health care field. You will also learn about the skills you will need to find a job that is both rewarding and enjoyable.

WORKING AS A PROFESSIONAL

What will you learn?

When you are finished with this section, you will be able to:

1. Discuss the qualities that contribute to a strong work ethic.
2. Describe what a "professional" looks like and how a professional behaves.
3. Understand the importance of taking proper care of yourself, and describe ways to keep yourself healthy, both physically and emotionally.
4. Define the words work ethic, professional, attitude, and hygiene.

Having a strong work ethic

Work ethic ▪▪▪ a person's attitude toward his or her work

A strong **work ethic** is what distinguishes an average employee from a great employee (Fig. 3-1). Two nursing assistants can have solid skills and be very good at getting their work done on time, but the nursing assistant with the strongest work ethic will be the one who enjoys the most success. What qualities does a person with a strong work ethic have, and how can one go about developing these qualities?

A professional attitude

Professional ▪▪▪ a person who has credentials, obtained through education and training, that enable him to become licensed or certified to practice a certain profession; also, a person who demonstrates a professional attitude

Attitude ▪▪▪ the side of ourselves that we display to the world, communicating outwardly how we feel about things

One definition of a **professional** is a person who has training that allows him or her to become licensed or certified to do a certain job. But even people who have jobs that do not require licensure or certification can behave in a professional manner. Being a professional also means having a positive **attitude**. A person's attitude is apparent from things he says (and the way he says them), the way he behaves, and the way he looks. Having a professional, positive attitude means that you are caring and compassionate toward your patients or residents and that you are committed to doing your job to the best of your ability at all times.

Punctuality

Being punctual means that you are on time or a little bit early. Many people are relying on you! Your patients or residents need you to help them. The staff members working the shift before yours need to go home so that they can attend to their families and other responsibilities, just as you need to attend to yours when you are at home.

Being late is sometimes unavoidable. But you can increase your chances of being on time by knowing how long it will take you to get to work and then adding 15 minutes to that travel time. Preparing ahead of time (for example, by packing your lunch and making sure your uniform is clean and ready to wear before you go to bed) can also make getting out the door easier when it is time to leave for work. Remember, chronic lateness is one of the main reasons employers take corrective action against nursing assistants.

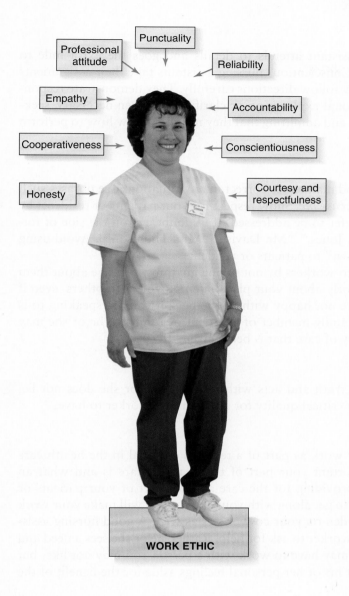

Professional attitude

Punctuality

Reliability

Empathy

Accountability

Cooperativeness

Conscientiousness

Honesty

Courtesy and respectfulness

WORK ETHIC

FIGURE ■ 3-1
Professionalism and a strong work ethic go hand in hand. Many qualities contribute to a strong work ethic.

Reliability

Reliability means that others can count on you to come to work every day as scheduled and to remain there during your entire shift. Have an emergency plan in place for transportation and childcare before the need arises, and try to keep yourself healthy to decrease your need to take sick days. Poor attendance is another major reason people lose their jobs.

Reliability also means that others can count on you to do your job well with minimal supervision. Your supervisor should not feel the need to look over your shoulder or check up on you to make sure your work has been finished.

Accountability

An accountable person accepts responsibility for his or her actions and the results of those actions. Being accountable means that you can accept criticism that is intended to help you improve, admit a mistake, and work to correct the situation.

Conscientiousness

A conscientious nursing assistant attends to details and goes the extra mile to complete a task with care. Conscientious nursing assistants take their assignments seriously and make sure they follow directions carefully. They demonstrate responsibility by asking for additional explanation or clarification when necessary, seeking help with difficult tasks, and admitting that they may not know how to perform a particular task.

Courtesy and respect

Being polite and having good manners is correct in any situation. Use phrases such as *please, thank you,* and *excuse me.* Show respect for your patients or residents by addressing them as they prefer to be addressed. If in doubt, err on the side of formality ("Dr. Smith," "Mrs. Jones," "Mr. Davis," "Miss Thomson"). Avoid using "baby talk" or "talking down" to patients or residents.

Show respect for your co-workers by not saying anything negative about them to others. Do not speak poorly about your place of employment to others, even if there are things that you are not happy with. If the person you are speaking to is a patient or resident (or a family member of a patient or resident), he or she may begin to question the quality of care that is being given.

Honesty

An honest person tells the truth and acts with integrity. He or she does not lie, cheat, or steal. Honesty is a critical quality for a health care worker to have.

Cooperativeness

Being able to cooperate, or work as part of a team, is essential in the health care field. Remember how important your part of the chain of care is and what an essential role you play in providing for the care and comfort of your patients or residents. Making an effort to get along with your co-workers will make your work easier and will ease the burden on your co-workers as well. A good nursing assistant does not wait for a co-worker to ask for help. Rather, he or she sees a need and offers a helping hand. You may have to work with a person you may not like, but a professional is able to put his or her personal feelings aside for the benefit of the patient or resident.

Empathy

Empathy means that you are able to try to imagine what it would feel like to be in another person's situation. There are times when other people will really try your patience, but if you think of how you would feel if you were in a similar situation, you may find that you are able to understand the offending behavior better. Empathy gives us another perspective and helps us to be kinder and more tolerant.

Maintaining a professional appearance

Others often judge us based on our appearance. To be considered a professional, you need to look the part! That means practicing good personal hygiene and dressing neatly and professionally (Guidelines Box 3-1). Good personal hygiene helps to

Hygiene ■■■ personal cleanliness

Guidelines Box 3-1   Guidelines for a Professional Appearance

What you do	Why you do it
Style your hair neatly and away from your face.	*Securing your hair away from your face keeps it away from equipment, out of your eyes, and out of your work. If your hair is not secured back, when you move your hair out of your eyes, any germs on your hands will be transferred to your hair and face.*
Keep your nails short and clean, with smoothly filed edges.	*Germs can hide under the tips of long nails. Long nails can also scratch a person's skin. Frequent hand washing can cause acrylic and false nails to lift, allowing water to become trapped underneath and leading to a fungal infection in the nailbed.*
Leave bracelets, necklaces, rings, and dangling earrings at home.	*A child or confused person might pull dangling earrings through your earlobes. Necklaces and bracelets get in the way and can get caught in equipment and broken. If you wear rings, germs can become trapped underneath them, which makes hand washing less effective. Rings can also scratch a person's skin when you are providing care.*
If you wear make-up, apply it lightly and tastefully.	*Wearing too much make-up or make-up that is too bright or too dark does not contribute to a professional appearance.*
If you wear cologne or perfume, it should be of a light fragrance and lightly applied.	*Many people are sensitive to fragrances and may find perfume or cologne that is of a strong scent or heavily applied offensive.*
Wear a clean, pressed uniform each day. Make sure that your shoes are polished.	*Attention to details, such as making sure that your uniform is wrinkle-free and your shoes are polished, says to others that you care about your appearance. A clean uniform is also essential for limiting the spread of infection.*
If you have a tattoo, try to select a uniform style that will conceal it. If you are thinking about getting a tattoo or body piercing, consider its location carefully.	*Many people feel that tattoos and body piercings make a person look less professional. Many employers now have dress code policies that require tattoos to be covered and limit the number of piercings an employee is allowed to have exposed.*
Practice good personal hygiene and grooming daily.	*Good personal hygiene helps to prevent breath and body odors and limits the spread of infection. In addition, if you care enough about yourself to keep yourself clean and neat, the people in your care will feel that you will do the same for them.*

prevent the spread of infection and promotes a neat, clean appearance. To practice good personal hygiene:

- Bathe daily and use a deodorant.
- Shampoo your hair regularly and treat dandruff or other scalp conditions.
- Keep your nails short and clean, with smoothly filed edges.
- Brush and floss your teeth, and use mouthwash. Visit a dentist regularly. Poor dental health can cause breath odors.
- If you are a man, shave daily, or keep facial hair neatly groomed and trimmed.
- Wear a clean, pressed uniform each day.
- Wash your hands often.

Staying healthy

To care for your patients or residents to the best of your ability, you must first care for yourself, both physically and emotionally. By taking proper care of yourself, you demonstrate that you are a professional who takes his or her responsibilities seriously.

Maintaining your physical health

The duties of a nursing assistant require much physical effort. You will be constantly lifting, bending, walking, and reaching as you perform your daily tasks at work. Your employer, your co-workers, your family, and especially your patients or residents rely on you to be able to do your duties. In addition to giving you more energy, staying physically fit keeps your body strong and allows you to avoid many types of job-related injuries. Guidelines for keeping your body in good physical condition are given in Guidelines Box 3-2.

Even the healthiest people occasionally get sick. If you are sick (especially if you have a fever), do not go to work. If you go to work with a contagious illness, you could give the illness to the people in your care. Many of the people in your care will have conditions that make it harder for them to fight off an infection if they are exposed to one (for example, they may be elderly or in poor general health). In this situation, the responsible thing to do is to notify your supervisor that you are ill and unable to come to work. Follow your facility's policy for calling in sick. This will allow your supervisor to find someone else to cover your shift.

Maintaining your emotional health

Caring for others is an emotionally demanding job, as well as a physically demanding one, for many reasons:

- Due to the shortage of health care workers, as well as a need to cut costs, many facilities are understaffed, which means that employees are often overworked.
- Not all patients or residents are happy, or grateful for the care they are receiving. Many people in need of care do not feel well and, as a result, may be difficult or hard to manage.

Guidelines Box 3-2   Guidelines for Staying Physically Healthy

What you do	Why you do it
Get enough sleep.	*Most people need an average of 6 to 8 hours of sleep to function properly. Not only does rest relax the muscles, it also relaxes the mind and allows you to think clearly. Too little rest can weaken your immune system, making you more likely to get infections, such as cold and flu viruses.*
Eat well-balanced, nutritious meals.	*A working body needs good nutrition. You need fuel for your muscles and your brain.*
Exercise regularly.	*Regular exercise gives you more strength and energy and keeps your heart and lungs healthy. In addition, regular exercise helps reduce the mental stress that sometimes goes along with intensely emotional jobs, such as those in the health care field.*
Do not smoke.	*Smoking causes the blood vessels in the body to narrow, reducing the flow of oxygen-carrying blood to the body's cells. Smoking is associated with serious diseases such as lung cancer, emphysema, and heart disease.*
Do not take recreational drugs. Limit the amount of alcohol you drink.	*Using recreational drugs or drinking too much alcohol can have many negative effects on your health. In addition, these substances can impair your ability to make good decisions, both on and off the job.*
Have a routine physical examination.	*Many chronic illnesses, such as high blood pressure and diabetes, go undetected until they have caused permanent damage to your body. Many types of cancers can be cured if detected early enough. Routine physical examinations can help you to detect problems early so that actions can be taken to correct them.*

■ As a health care worker, you will have to face the death of some of your patients or residents. This can be difficult, especially in situations where you have had a chance to develop a relationship with the person and his or her family members.

Fortunately, there are actions you can take to help keep your emotions in check while you are on the job and prevent emotional burnout. Some of these actions are listed in Guidelines Box 3-3.

Guidelines Box 3-3   Guidelines for Staying Emotionally Healthy

What you do	Why you do it
Maintain your physical health.	*Physical activity relieves mental and emotional stress.*
Schedule time for yourself.	*Most of us are not just caregivers in the workplace; we are caregivers at home as well. It is important to make time for yourself, to do what you like to do, in order to avoid feeling overwhelmed by your responsibilities at home and at work.*
Take advantage of counseling services offered by your employer or confide in a clergy member.	*Talking to a professional can help you to manage work-related stress and define your feelings and beliefs about difficult subjects, such as death and dying.*
When a situation becomes particularly "heated" at work, take a physical and emotional break. Ask someone to relieve you, and take a walk outside to calm down.	*When we reach our limits, we may say or do something we regret later. Acting in frustration or anger can put your professional relationships at risk and may even cause you to harm a patient or resident. Physically removing yourself from the situation can give you a new perspective and the opportunity to calm down before going back to work.*
Ask to be assigned to different work areas or to different patients or residents occasionally.	*New situations and challenges help to prevent boredom and burnout.*

Putting it all together!

- Regardless of the level of education, certification, or experience a health care professional has, professionalism is all about exhibiting the right attitude, to co-workers, patients or residents, and visitors.

- A person with a strong work ethic can be depended on and trusted; treats others with kindness, respect, and compassion; and is committed to doing his or her job to the best of his or her ability at all times.

- Personal hygiene promotes a professional image and helps to prevent the spread of infection. In the health care field, many of the traits we have come to associate with a professional image are related to maintaining safety and health.

- To care for your patients or residents to the best of your ability, you must first care for yourself. Staying physically fit keeps your body strong and helps to prevent many types of job-related injuries. Taking steps to maintain your emotional health helps to prevent emotional burnout.

FINDING A JOB

What will you learn?

When you are finished with this section, you will be able to:

1. Describe questions a person should consider before beginning a job search.
2. List places to search for job openings.
3. Describe how to complete a job application.
4. Describe ways to make a good first impression during an interview.
5. Define the words résumé, reference list, and interview.

The health care field is one of the most rapidly growing areas in industry, and the trend is expected to continue. People who are trained to work as nursing assistants are in great demand. Your goal is to find a job situation in which you will be happy and professionally fulfilled. To do that, you need to take a methodical approach to looking for a job.

Think about your ideal job

Before you begin the process of searching for job openings, completing applications, and going on interviews, it is important that you take time to explore what you really want from your employment and what you will be able to offer to your employer. Some questions to consider are shown in Figure 3-2.

Search for job openings

Once you have some specific goals in mind, there are many places to search for job openings. Some examples are:

- Classified ads in the local newspaper
- Telephone directories (look under listings such as "retirement communities and homes," "home health services," and "hospitals" for names of local places that might hire nursing assistants)
- Internet sites dedicated to helping people find jobs
- Your school's job placement service
- Bulletin boards in the facility where you are receiving clinical training
- Friends and colleagues

Prepare your paperwork

Before applying for a job, you should prepare two key documents: a résumé and a reference list. You may also wish to prepare a cover letter.

Résumé ■■■ a brief document that gives a possible employer general information about a job candidate's education and work experience

Reference list ■■■ a list of three or four people who would be willing to talk to a potential employer about a job candidate's abilities

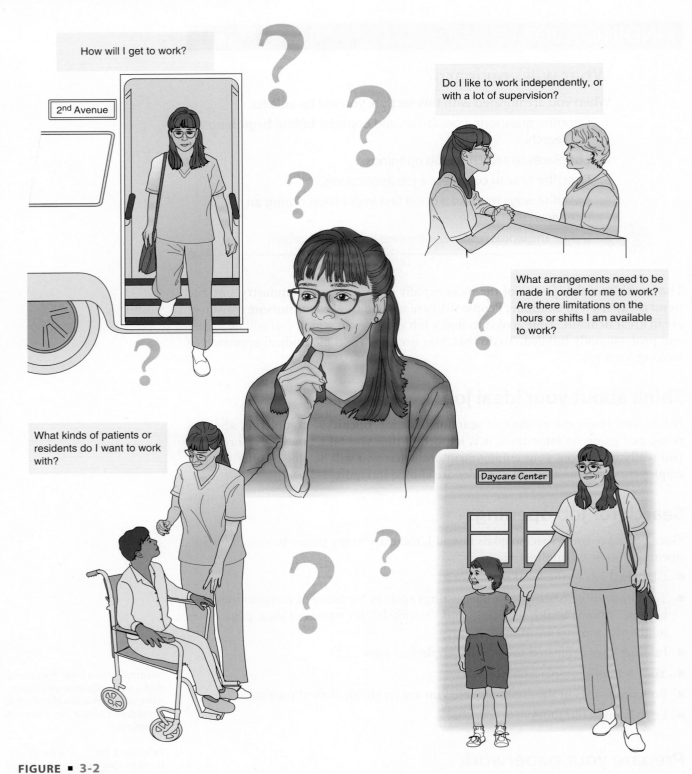

How will I get to work?

2nd Avenue

Do I like to work independently, or with a lot of supervision?

What arrangements need to be made in order for me to work? Are there limitations on the hours or shifts I am available to work?

What kinds of patients or residents do I want to work with?

Daycare Center

FIGURE ■ 3-2
The first step to finding a job is thinking about what sort of situation best fits your personality, lifestyle, and interests.

Résumés

Type or print your résumé using a computer on white or off-white paper. Include only facts, and try to keep your résumé to one page, if at all possible. Your résumé should include:

- Your full name, address, telephone number, and, if you have one, e-mail address.
- A short objective or career goal.
- A history of your education (list the schools you attended most recently first, and for each school, include the dates you attended the school and the degree you graduated with).
- An employment history (list each of your previous employers, and for each employer, include the dates that you worked, your job title, and your primary job duties).

There is some information that should never be included on a résumé, including your age, marital status, weight, religion, sexual preference, and whether or not you have children (or are planning to have them). This information should not matter to an employer who is considering you as an employee.

Reference lists

When considering people to include on your reference list, think about people who know you well and have worked with you in a professional capacity, such as your teachers, co-workers, and previous supervisors. Before listing a person as a reference, make sure you have the person's permission to do so. After a person has agreed to be your reference, make sure you have accurate contact information for that person, including his or her full name and title (if any), a current and complete address, and a telephone number. Type your reference list on a sheet of paper that matches your résumé.

Cover letters

You may also want to prepare a cover letter to send out with your résumé and reference list. A cover letter is written as a way of introducing yourself to a potential employer. Your résumé contains information about your education, training, and experience, but a cover letter goes beyond the straight facts. A cover letter says, "Hello, this is why I want to work for your organization, and this is why I am the best person for the job." Your cover letter should be fairly short and typed or printed using a computer on white or off-white paper. Pay special attention to your grammar and spelling.

Put in applications

The next step is to apply for jobs that you are interested in. You can visit facilities where you are interested in working and ask to complete a job application. A job application is a form that employers use to obtain basic information about you, such as which position you are applying for, how you can be reached, and what shifts you can work. The application form will also require you to provide information about your education, your work history, and the reasons you left your previous job. The job application is a legal document, and your signature at the bottom states that all the information is true and accurate. Always be honest when filling out a job application. An employer who finds out that you lied about any information on the application form has grounds to fire you without notice.

Usually, when you go to an organization to complete a job application, the receptionist at the main desk will give you the application to complete. When completing the job application, use blue or black ink and write clearly. Have your résumé and reference list with you. Many employers request copies of these along with your completed job application. In addition, having these documents with you will make it easier to fill out the job application accurately.

When you go to complete your job application, dress appropriately. Some facilities may choose to interview you at that time, especially if there is an opening. Appropriate dress means "clean and neat." Even if you do not interview, this will be the first impression you make on a possible employer.

Ask for an appointment for an interview when you submit your résumé, reference list, and completed application. Some facilities will make the appointment at this time. Others may want to review your résumé and application and call you for an appointment at a later date. If you have not heard from a potential employer in 1 week's time, it is appropriate to call and ask about the status of your application. A follow-up call shows a potential employer that you have initiative and are interested in the job.

Go on interviews

Interview ■■■ a meeting between an employer and a potential employee during which information is exchanged regarding the organization, the job, and the potential employee's qualifications for the job

During the interview, the interviewer will be trying to determine whether you are the right person for the job. The interview is also a chance for *you* to learn more about the employer and the position in an effort to determine whether they are right for you. Being properly prepared for the interview will allow you to gather as much information about the organization and the job as possible during the interview so that you can make a decision about the job if it is offered to you. In addition, being properly prepared can make all the difference in how a potential employer views your potential! Your résumé and application contain all of the "hard" facts about your education and experience, but you are the one responsible for persuading the interviewer of your interest in the job, dedication to your profession, and abilities.

Before going to the interview, make a list of questions you would like answers to, and refer to this list during the interview. This shows that you are interested in the position and are taking the opportunity to interview seriously. Some questions you might want to ask are shown in Box 3-1. You should also think about the answers to questions the interviewer might ask you so that you can be prepared to answer them. Some of these questions are shown in Box 3-2.

You are interviewing for a job in the health care setting, so help the interviewer see you as a part of his or her staff. Present yourself as a well-groomed professional (see Guidelines Box 3-1). Make sure your clothing is pressed and that all repairs, such as replacing missing buttons or fixing loose seams, have been taken care of before the interview. Your shoes should be clean and polished. If you are a man, wear slacks (not jeans), a button-down shirt or a polo shirt, and a belt, and possibly a sport jacket if the weather is cool. A tie is optional. If you are a woman, wear a skirt (or dress slacks) and a blouse or a simple dress. Wear stockings, and make sure that the hem length of your skirt or dress is modest.

Box 3-1   Questions You Might Want to Ask the Interviewer

- "What are the major responsibilities or duties of the position? May I have a copy of the job description?"

- "May I see the unit where I will be working and meet the person who will be supervising me?"

- "What do you think nursing assistants like best about working here? Least?"

- "How many nursing assistants staff each unit?"

- "When would I be eligible for a performance evaluation, and what are the standards I will be evaluated against?"

- "What qualities are you looking for in a nursing assistant?"

- "What opportunities exist for career growth and furthering my education?"

Box 3-2   Questions that an Interviewer Might Want to Ask You

- "Tell me about yourself. Why did you become a nursing assistant?"

- "What part of your last job did you like the most? The least?"

- "Why are you leaving your current job?" (or, "Why did you leave your last job?")

- "What are you looking for in a manager?"

- "How do you describe your work habits?"

- "How do you set priorities?"

- "How do you handle yourself under stress?"

- "How do you handle problems with patients or co-workers?"

- "Tell me about a specific situation that interfered with your ability to do your job, and how you handled it."

- "What is the most satisfying workday you have had this year? Why?"

- "Do you have a mentor? What have you learned from this person?"

- "Who in your life would you consider to be 'successful'? Why?"

- "What do you consider to be your greatest strength? Your greatest weakness?"

- "Where do you want to go with your career? What steps have you taken to achieve your goal?"

- "What is it about our organization that appeals to you?"

Carrying a small notebook containing the questions you want to ask during the interview and a copy of your résumé, reference list, and your certified nursing assistant certification or registration looks very professional. Do not chew gum during the interview, and make sure your cellular phone is turned off. You only have one chance to make a first impression, so make it a good one!

Give yourself adequate time to get to the interview. Ideally, you will arrive a few minutes early. After being introduced to the interviewer, shake his or her hand and take a seat when you are invited to do so. Do not address the interviewer by his or her first name unless the interviewer specifically asks you to. Thank the person for the opportunity to interview at the beginning of the interview.

During the interview process, sit up straight and try not to fidget. You might be nervous, but try to appear as confident and comfortable as you can. Maintain good eye contact during the interview and speak clearly. Try to answer questions concisely yet completely; it is best if you can strike a balance between listening and talking. If you do not know the answer to a question, simply say that you do not know—most interviewers are quick to recognize bluffing.

At the end of the interview, the interviewer will usually give you an opportunity to ask any questions that you may have. Now is the time to refer to your list! Asking questions of your own indicates that you have an active interest in making sure that you are a good fit for the job and the organization. When the interview is over, thank the interviewer again for his or her time and for considering you for the position. If the interviewer did not mention when you can expect to hear from him or her regarding the position, ask. Then leave! The interview is over, and there is nothing left to do but write a thank-you note.

You should write a short thank-you note within 1 day of interviewing for the position, thanking the interviewer for considering you for the position and briefly explaining why you are excited about the possibility of working for his or her organization. You may hand write your thank-you note on a plain note card or type it.

Accept an offer

When someone calls to offer you a job, you may be ready to accept it right away. Or, you might need time to think about it. If so, it is acceptable to ask the person if you can call him or her back with an answer within a day or so. If you have not heard from the organization you interviewed with within the amount of time specified at the close of the interview, it is appropriate to follow up with a telephone call. Even if this job did not work out, another one will. Just keep trying!

Chances are, you will accept many different jobs over the course of your career. You may need to leave a job when a better opportunity comes along or because of a change in your personal circumstances (such as a move to a new area). You may leave a job to stay at home with your children or go back to school. When leaving a job, give your employer at least 2 weeks' notice so that arrangements can be made

Getting the perfect job is just the beginning. Keeping the job and growing professionally are just as important. Remember the qualities that a person with a strong work ethic possesses? By demonstrating these qualities daily at work, you will quickly become a valuable member of the health care team. You will be open to learning new information and skills, and your patients or residents will certainly benefit from your professional growth and dedication to providing quality care.

to cover your shifts. Write a letter stating your desire to leave the job and thanking your present employer for the opportunity to work at the organization. Make sure you leave in good standing because you never know when you may need a good job reference from that employer or actually find that you really want your old job back!

Putting it all together!

- Thinking about the type of job you want helps to give direction to your job search.

- Applying and interviewing for jobs can be a time-consuming process that requires a lot of effort. However, by taking the time to prepare, you increase your chances of finding a situation in which you will be happy and satisfied with your work.

What did you learn?

Multiple Choice

Select the single best answer for each of the following questions.

1. A short, precise document with information about you, your work experience, and your education is called a:
   a. Minimum Data Set (MDS)
   b. Résumé
   c. Reference
   d. Cover letter

2. All of the following information should be included on your résumé, except for your:
   a. Name
   b. Address
   c. Employment history
   d. Religion

3. Which one of the following is a legal document used when applying for a job?
   a. Résumé
   b. Cover letter
   c. Reference list
   d. Application

4. The chance for a potential employer to meet you personally occurs during the:
   a. Application process
   b. Interview process
   c. Job posting process
   d. Reference checking process

5. A nursing assistant can promote his or her physical health by doing all of the following except:
   a. Eating well-balanced meals
   b. Getting plenty of rest
   c. Smoking and drinking socially
   d. Attending aerobics classes

6. A nursing assistant's personal cleanliness is referred to as:
   a. Sanitization
   b. Neatness
   c. Hygiene
   d. Fashion

7. Qualities that characterize a good work ethic include all of the following except:
   a. Reliability
   b. Punctuality
   c. Honesty
   d. Tardiness

8. What type of a nursing assistant accepts responsibility for his or her actions?
   a. An accountable nursing assistant
   b. A respectful nursing assistant
   c. A courteous nursing assistant
   d. A punctual nursing assistant

9. What type of a nursing assistant is able to imagine what it would feel like to be in another person's situation?
   a. A creative nursing assistant
   b. An empathetic nursing assistant
   c. An experienced nursing assistant
   d. An honest nursing assistant

10. What type of a nursing assistant can be counted on to come to work every day?
    a. A punctual nursing assistant
    b. A nursing assistant with access to public transportation
    c. A reliable nursing assistant
    d. An ethical nursing assistant

11. What type of nursing assistant has a professional attitude?
    a. A nursing assistant who acts smarter than the other nursing assistants
    b. A nursing assistant who is certified
    c. A nursing assistant who is committed to doing his or her best at all times
    d. A nursing assistant who is always late to work

Stop and Think!

Imagine that you have just completed your nursing assistant training and taken the state test. While you are waiting for your test results, you decide to begin reading job postings to see what opportunities are available. At this point, you are considering several options. You are excited about beginning your career in the health care field, and you are anxious to get into the workforce and put your new skills to use. However, you think that you might also want to continue your education and become either a licensed practical nurse (LPN) or a registered nurse (RN) someday. What sorts of organizations may be looking for nursing assistants in your community? How could working as a nursing assistant now help you to further define your career goals?

STOP **Stop and Think!**

Your best friend Martha is also a nursing assistant at the long-term care facility where you work. She has a very difficult time managing her personal life and her professional life. Many times, Martha has asked you to clock her in when you get to work so that your supervisors will not see that she is late. This makes you uncomfortable, but you do not want to lose Martha's friendship. What should you do?

CHAPTER 4

A nursing assistant talks with one of her residents.

Communication Skills

ommunicating—that is, sharing and receiving information—is something that you have to do every day. In this chapter, you will learn skills and tactics that you can use to enhance your ability to communicate. We will also review some of the tools that are used by members of the health care team to ensure that important information is available to all who are involved with the care of a patient or resident.

INTRODUCTION TO COMMUNICATION

What will you learn?

When you are finished with this section, you will be able to:

1. Understand what communication is.
2. Discuss why it is important for a nursing assistant to be able to communicate effectively.
3. Describe the two major forms of communication and give examples of each.
4. Discuss techniques that promote effective communication.
5. Define the words communication, verbal communication, and nonverbal communication.

The key to understanding what communication is lies within the word "exchange." If you exchange gifts with another person, you give that person a gift, and, in return, you receive one back. Communicating is not just about telling someone something (giving information). It is also about listening and observing (receiving information). For communication to be effective, all of the people who are involved must actively participate in the exchange of information (Fig. 4-1).

There are two major forms of communication, verbal communication and nonverbal communication. Verbal communication uses words, either spoken or written, to exchange information. Examples of verbal communication include telephone conversations, written notes and memos, e-mail and text messages, and ASL (American Sign Language) that is used to communicate with people who are deaf. Verbal communication tends to be more direct—when we use language to express

Communication ▪▪▪ the exchange of information

Verbal communication ▪▪▪ a way of communicating that uses written or spoken language

Nonverbal communication ▪▪▪ a way of communicating that uses facial expressions, gestures, and body language, instead of written or spoken language

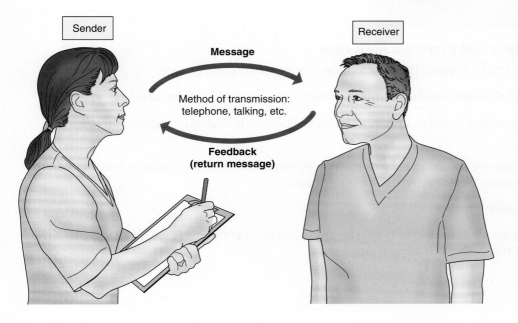

Sender

Receiver

Message

Method of transmission: telephone, talking, etc.

Feedback (return message)

FIGURE ▪ 4-1

Communication involves at least two people, a *sender* and a *receiver*. The sender is the person with information to share and the receiver is the person for whom the information is intended. The sender delivers the information in the form of a *message*, which the receiver may or may not understand. Through *feedback*, or a return message, the receiver lets the sender know whether the message was received and understood. Note that as information is transmitted back and forth, the sender and the receiver switch roles.

a thought, it is usually with the intent of giving specific information to another person. Nonverbal communication, on the other hand, tends to be more indirect. Being aware of nonverbal cues can give you a better understanding of what other people are truly feeling and thinking.

As a nursing assistant, you must be a successful communicator, both as a sender and a receiver of information, with both those you care for and your co-workers. You will use your communication skills to:

- Comfort, reassure, and teach your patients or residents
- Share information about changes in your patients' or residents' health status with other members of the health care team
- Accept or decline assigned tasks and seek additional clarification about how to do those tasks as necessary

Tips on how to be a good communicator are given in Box 4-1.

Box 4-1 How to Be a Good Communicator

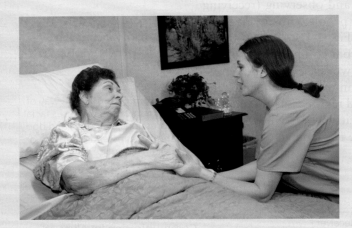

When you are the sender, make sure your message is clear

- Think about what you want to say. Present the information in a logical, organized way.

- If your message is written, make sure your handwriting is neat and your spelling is accurate.

- Speak clearly at a normal pace, and avoid mumbling. Unless the person is hearing impaired, there is no reason to raise your voice.

- Use words that the person you are speaking to understands. When appropriate, use simple, common words in place of more technical words. If necessary, use an interpreter.

- Face the person you are speaking to.

- Make sure that the person you are speaking to is able to physically receive the message. For example, if the person wears a hearing aid, make sure it is turned on.

Box 4-1   How to Be a Good Communicator (Continued)

When you are the receiver, be a good listener

- Focus your attention on the speaker.

- Sit down and do not appear rushed or in a hurry.

- Make eye contact with the speaker.

- Do not interrupt or try to finish the speaker's sentences.

Learn techniques for encouraging people to talk

- Ask open-ended questions instead of "yes/no" questions. For example, instead of asking "Did you have breakfast this morning?," ask "What did you have for breakfast this morning?"

- Rephrase what the person says to you. For example, if a resident says that she feels sad and lonely, instead of asking "Why?," say "You're feeling sad and lonely?" This invites the person to talk more about what she is feeling.

- Observe for and ask questions about nonverbal signals the person may be sending.

- Remember the value of silence and a comforting touch.

Provide and seek feedback

- When you are the receiver, ask questions and repeat information back to the sender so that he or she knows that his or her message was received and understood.

- When you are the sender, seek feedback from the receiver to make sure that he or she understood your message. This is always important, but especially so when the person may be embarrassed about an inability to understand you (for example, if the person has hearing loss or speaks a language that is different from yours).

- Observe for nonverbal cues that indicate that the receiver did not understand your message. For example, the person may be nodding his or her head but looking confused.

Avoid behaviors that block effective communication

- Avoid being judgmental. A person who is judgmental forms quick opinions about whether or not another person is right or wrong. A judgmental attitude can be revealed through body language or comments you make and indicates to the other person that you do not respect his or her thoughts, beliefs, or feelings.

- Avoid assuming that another person knows what you are thinking. Instead, keep others informed about what you have done and what you expect them to do.

- Avoid "tuning out" others. Always listen carefully.

- Avoid negative body language, such as tapping your fingers or foot impatiently, constantly looking at your watch or toward the door, crossing your arms, and rolling your eyes.

- Avoid using slang or foul language.

Putting it all together!

- For communication to be effective, all of the people who are involved must actively participate in the exchange of information.
- The two major forms of communication are verbal and nonverbal. Verbal communication involves the use of language, either spoken or written. Nonverbal communication gives information through the use of facial expressions, gestures, or body language.
- Nursing assistants must be effective communicators, both as senders and receivers of information, with both co-workers and people who are receiving care.
- Listening is one of the most important communication skills, especially in the health care field. Speaking clearly, asking open-ended questions, and using appropriate body language are other ways to ensure effective communication.

COMMUNICATING WITH PEOPLE WITH SPECIAL NEEDS

What will you learn?

When you are finished with this section, you will be able to:

1. Discuss situations that might affect a person's ability to communicate effectively.
2. Describe how a nursing assistant can assist with communication in these situations.

Communicating with a person who speaks a language different from yours

Some of your patients or residents may not speak the same language that you do. When caring for a person who speaks a foreign language:

- Use hand gestures or a picture board (Fig. 4-2) to communicate very basic ideas.
- You may need to use an interpreter to avoid misunderstandings.

Communicating with a person who has hearing loss

You may care for patients or residents who have been deaf since birth or who have become completely or partially deaf as a result of a disorder that affects the ear. In addition, many older people gradually lose the ability to hear high-pitched sounds as part of the normal aging process. When this occurs, the older person has trouble

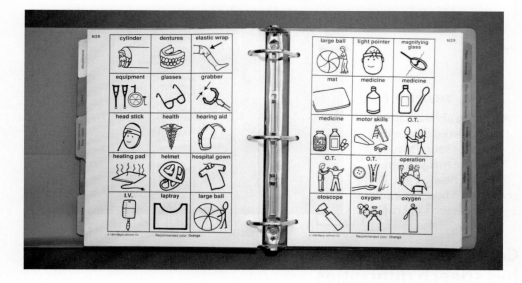

FIGURE ■ **4-2**

A picture board is often useful when trying to communicate on a basic level with someone who speaks a different language, is hearing impaired, or has a developmental disability.

telling the difference between similar-sounding high-pitched sounds like *th* and *s*. This can lead to frequent misunderstandings. When caring for a person with hearing loss:

- Face the person when you are speaking to him or her. This gives the person a clear view of your mouth, which is helpful if the person lip-reads. Avoid chewing gum or speaking unusually fast because these actions can make it hard for the person to read your lips. If the person needs glasses, make sure he or she is wearing them so that your lips can be seen clearly.

- Use a note pad to write down important questions or directions so that the person can read them.

- Consider learning sign language or using a sign language interpreter (Fig. 4-3).

- If a person who uses a hearing aid (Fig. 4-4) seems unable to hear you, make sure the hearing aid is turned on and that the volume is turned up high enough. If the hearing aid still does not seem to be working, check the batteries to see whether they need to be replaced. You will learn more about how to care for and operate hearing aids in Chapter 20.

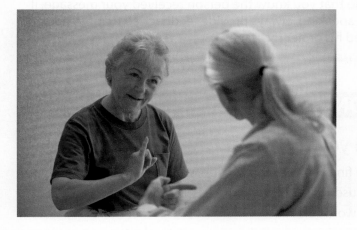

FIGURE ■ **4-3**

Sign language is a form of verbal communication used by many people with significant hearing loss.

Will & Deni McIntyre/Photo Researchers, Inc.

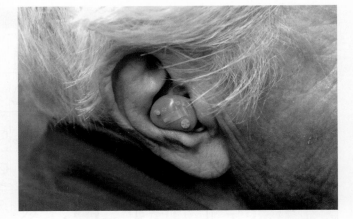

FIGURE ■ 4-4

A hearing aid is a battery-powered device that makes sounds louder. There are many different styles of hearing aid. The style shown here fits inside the person's ear canal.

Communicating with a person who has speech difficulties

There are many reasons why a person might have trouble speaking clearly. People who are completely deaf often do not speak clearly. A person who has had a stroke may lose the ability to form sounds into meaningful words. Surgical procedures affecting the mouth or vocal cords can make it difficult or impossible for a person to speak. So can medical devices, such as breathing tubes. When caring for a person who has trouble speaking:

- Ask "yes/no" questions when all you need is basic information.
- If you cannot understand what the person is saying, please tell the person that you did not understand and look for other ways to help the person communicate. For example, you might offer the person a note pad so that she can write down what she needs to tell you or a picture board so that she can point to what she needs.

Putting it all together!

- Special situations that may affect communication include language differences, hearing loss, and conditions that affect a person's ability to speak.
- When communicating with a person who has special needs, it is especially important to practice the good communication techniques described in Box 4-1. If the person has trouble hearing or understanding the language, always seek feedback so that you know the person received your message. If the person has trouble speaking, always provide feedback so that the person knows that you received his or her message.

RESOLVING CONFLICTS

What will you learn?

When you are finished with this section, you will be able to:

1. Identify causes of conflict and discuss ways of resolving conflicts.
2. Define the word **conflict**.

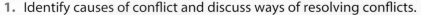

Conflict is common in the health care field because health care is a people-oriented, emotional business. Patients and residents are sick, hurting, confused, and frightened. Family members feel helpless and sad. Staff members are often stressed by the emotional and physical demands of their work. As a result, conflicts may arise between a member of the health care team and a patient or resident, between two patients or residents, or between two members of the health care team. Conflict makes the people directly involved, as well as those around them, uncomfortable. If you find yourself involved in a conflict, take steps to resolve the problem quickly and professionally (Box 4-2).

Conflict ▪▪▪ discord resulting from differences between people; can occur when one person is unable to understand or accept another's ideas or beliefs

Putting it all together!

- Getting along with other people, although it is a very important part of your job, can sometimes be the hardest part of your job.

- Good communication is essential to preventing conflict, as well as helping to resolve it.

- A conflict that affects the quality of the care you provide must not be allowed to continue! If you find yourself involved in a conflict, remember what it means to be a professional and take appropriate steps to resolve the issue.

Box 4-2   How to Resolve a Conflict

- Ask to speak privately with the person you have a conflict with. Because the two of you may be able to resolve your disagreement on your own, try this approach before involving a supervisor. Remain polite and professional, and thank the person for his or her time.

- During your conversation, focus on the specific area of conflict. Do not focus on how you feel about the other person or how you think he or she should have acted under the circumstances.

- Be specific about what you understand the problem to be. Express why you are upset, but avoid being accusatory. For example, instead of saying "You really hurt my feelings by what you said the other day," say, "I am bothered by what you said the other day." This allows you to take responsibility for your emotions while allowing the other person to explain his or her side of the story.

- Be prepared to hear how the other person may feel toward you or the problem, even if it is not pleasant. Perhaps you were the one who was initially misunderstood.

- Be gracious enough to apologize for misunderstanding the other person or for being the one who was misunderstood.

- Ask the other person for ideas about how to resolve the conflict. His or her suggestions might surprise you!

- Sometimes it is necessary to "agree to disagree." People with differing opinions and beliefs can focus on things they have in common, such as caring about the patient's or resident's well-being, and still disagree on certain issues. Learning to respect others' beliefs is part of being professional.

- If you cannot resolve a conflict on your own, seek the advice of your supervisor.

USING THE TELEPHONE

What will you learn?

When you are finished with this section, you will be able to:

1. Demonstrate proper telephone communication skills.
2. Explain in general terms what information a nursing assistant is not permitted to provide or receive via the telephone.

As a nursing assistant, you will usually be required to answer the telephone, either at the nursing station or in a patient's or resident's room. The way you handle yourself on the telephone reflects directly on your facility. General policies for how to use the telephone properly are given in Box 4-3.

Box 4-3   How to Use the Telephone

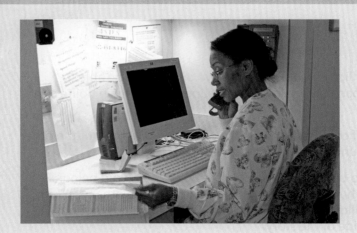

- Answer the telephone promptly, within the first three rings.

- Answer with a pleasant greeting, such as "Good morning" or "Good afternoon."

- Identify yourself by name and title and by your unit or floor according to facility policy: "3 West; Mary Smith, CNA, speaking."

- Because the caller obviously needs something (otherwise, he or she would not be calling), ask "How may I help you?"

- Know how to perform basic functions using your facility's telephone system, such as how to transfer a call or place a caller on hold.

- If you must place a caller on hold, ask his or her permission first ("May I put you on hold for a minute?"). Be aware of the length of time a caller has been on hold; if the time becomes excessive (more than 5 minutes), ask the caller if he or she wants to continue to hold, leave a message, or call back later.

- If the person the caller wants to speak to is unavailable, offer to take a message. When taking a telephone message, be sure to write down the date and time of the call, the name of the caller, a telephone number where the caller can be reached, and your name. Write clearly, and ask the caller to spell his or her name if you are not sure how to spell it. Be sure to deliver the message to the person for whom it was intended.

- A nursing assistant is not to take doctor's orders or receive or give results of diagnostic tests. Calls of this nature should be handled by a nurse.

- Know your facility's policy regarding what information can be provided over the telephone and

Box 4-3   How to Use the Telephone (Continued)

to whom. The Health Insurance Portability and Accountability Act (HIPAA), discussed in Chapter 2, specifically regulates who may be given information about a person in a health care facility. In general, callers seeking information about a patient or resident should be referred to the nurse.

- Do not use the telephone at the nurse's station to make or receive personal calls. Personal calls should be made from a pay phone or your own cellular phone, while you are on break or at lunch. Never tie up a telephone used for health care communication by using it for personal business.

Putting it all together!

- Using proper telephone etiquette improves communication and promotes a professional image.
- Confidentiality is of concern when the telephone is used as a means of communication. Protect yourself, your employer, and your patients or residents by being aware of your facility's policies with regard to telephone use.

> *Nursing assistants are an important link between the patient or resident and other members of the health care team. The nursing assistant is often the first member of the health care team to become aware of a change in a patient's or resident's condition that could be a sign of something serious.*

COMMUNICATION AMONG MEMBERS OF THE HEALTH CARE TEAM

What will you learn?

When you are finished with this section, you will be able to:

1. Explain why a nursing assistant is often considered the "eyes and ears" of the health care team.
2. Discuss the methods of reporting and recording information in a health care setting.
3. Define the words observations, objective data, signs, subjective data, symptom, reporting, recording, medical record (chart), and Kardex.

Observation ■■■ something that you notice about the patient or resident, typically related to a change in the person's physical or mental condition

Making observations

The amount of time you will spend with your patients or residents, combined with the duties you are responsible for performing daily (e.g., bathing, feeding, ambulating, toileting), means that you may notice things about your patients or residents that other health care team members may overlook. These things you notice are

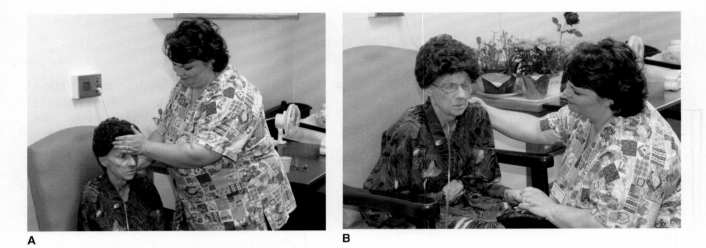

A **B**

FIGURE ▪ 4-5

(A) Objective data. When you collect objective data, you obtain information by using one of your five senses. Here, the nursing assistant is feeling the resident's forehead to find out whether the skin is hot and dry or cool and clammy. Other examples of objective data include a person's vital sign measurements, the smell and color of a person's urine, the sound of a person's breathing, and the color and condition of a person's skin. **(B) Subjective data.** Subjective data are information that you get second-hand. This nursing assistant knows that her resident is experiencing stomach pain because the resident is describing it to her, not because she detected the resident's pain using one of her five senses. Other examples of subjective data include a person's complaint of a headache, feeling nauseated, or feeling dizzy.

Objective ▪▪▪ information that is obtained directly, through measurements or by using one of the five senses (sight, smell, taste, hearing, touch)

Subjective ▪▪▪ information that cannot be objectively measured or assessed

Signs ▪▪▪ Objective evidence of disease, based on data that are obtained directly, through measurements or by using one of the five senses

Symptoms ▪▪▪ Subjective evidence of disease, based on data that cannot be measured or observed first-hand, such as a patient's or resident's complaint of pain

Reporting ▪▪▪ the spoken exchange of information between health care team members

Recording ▪▪▪ communicating information about a patient or resident to other health care team members in written form; sometimes called *charting or documenting*

called observations. Your observations may be based either on objective data or subjective data (Fig. 4-5). Objective data—such as an elevated temperature, a rash, or a low urine output—are called signs. Subjective data—such as pain, nausea, or dizziness—are called symptoms.

Reporting and recording

Nursing assistants use two methods of communicating observations about their patients or residents and documenting the care provided so that other health care team members are kept "in-the-know." These methods are reporting and recording (Fig. 4-6).

Reporting

Nursing assistants use reporting to communicate information to the nurse throughout the shift. Reporting is also used when shifts change to keep the staff members who are just arriving at work aware of all the information that is necessary to ensure a smooth continuation of care for the patient or resident. Throughout this text, specific observations that need to be reported to the nurse immediately are highlighted as "Tell the Nurse!" notes.

When reporting, remember to be a good communicator (see Box 4-1). Make sure the information that you are reporting is accurate—refer to the patient or resident by name and room number, and if you are reporting measurements, such as vital signs, write the numbers down so that you do not forget them or report them incorrectly. Report your observations in an orderly, concise manner. Avoid adding information that is not relevant to what you are trying to communicate. Use correct

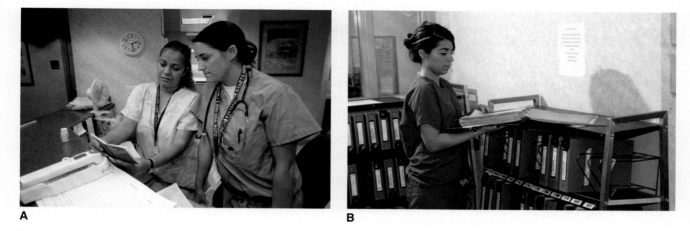

A   **B**

FIGURE ■ 4-6

(A) Reporting is the spoken exchange of information between health care team members. Here, a nursing assistant is reporting a change in one of her resident's vital signs to the nurse. **(B) Recording** is communicating information about a patient or resident to other health care team members in written form. Here, a nursing assistant checks a resident's medical record.

terminology when reporting, and make sure the person you are reporting to gives you feedback so that you know he or she received the information and will act on it.

Recording

MEDICAL RECORD (CHART) The medical record is usually organized in sections with specific forms contained in each section. Some of these forms provide general information about the patient or resident. Others are specific to a particular health care department. The forms used may vary depending on the type of facility or health care agency. Table 4-1 describes some of the forms that are typically found in a medical record.

Your employer will have specific policies about whether or not nursing assistants are allowed to record information in the medical record. If you are allowed to record information in the medical record, remember that the medical record is a formal record of the care the person received from the health care facility, and it can be retrieved at any time and used in a court of law as evidence in a lawsuit. For this reason, it is important to follow the guidelines in Guidelines Box 4-1 for recording.

The information contained in a person's medical record is considered confidential and is only to be read by members of the health care team who are directly involved in the care of that person and need access to the information in the record to provide that care. For example, although a custodial worker is part of the health care team, he or she does not need access to the information in the medical record to perform his or her duties. Therefore, custodial workers generally do not have access to patients' or residents' charts.

Some facilities will use computers for recording. In computerized recording, the person's medical record is maintained by entering data into a computer in response to the computer's prompts, rather than by filling in a paper form. To protect the patient's or resident's confidentiality, each user of the computer is assigned a password, which permits the user to have access to certain patients' or residents' medical records. Your facility will have specific policies—mandated by the Health Insurance Portability and Accountability Act (HIPAA)— regarding computer use

TELL THE NURSE !

In general, you need to report the following types of observations to the nurse immediately:

- Observations that suggest a change in the patient's or resident's condition
- Observations regarding the patient's or resident's response to a new treatment or therapy
- A patient's or resident's complaints of pain or discomfort
- A patient's or resident's refusal of treatment
- A patient's or resident's request for clergy

Medical record ■■■ a legal document where information about a patient's or resident's current condition, the measures that have been taken by the medical and nursing staff to diagnose and treat the condition, and the patient's or resident's response to the treatment and care provided is recorded; also called a *medical chart*

TABLE 4-1	Forms Found in a Typical Medical Record (Chart)
FORM	**PURPOSE**
Admission sheet	Contains standard information about the person such as the person's name, address, age, gender, insurance information, emergency notification information, and advance directive information.
Medical history	Lists a person's previous surgeries and medical conditions, current medications, allergies, and current medical diagnosis
Nursing history	Contains information about the person's needs as they relate to nursing care
Physician's order sheet	Used to order diagnostic tests and treatments and to specify dietary orders or activity status
Medication administration record (MAR)	Lists the medications ordered for the patient or resident, as well as the dose and time at which they are to be given; also used to record when medications were given and by whom
Physician's progress notes	Contains observations about the person's responses to treatments
Narrative nurse's notes	Used to document the person's complaints (symptoms) and the actions taken by the nursing staff in response to them
Graphic sheet	Contains information that is gathered routinely, such as vital signs, the frequency of urination and bowel movements, and food and fluid intake

and confidentiality. Make sure that you are familiar with these policies, and follow them carefully.

Kardex ■■■ a card file that contains condensed versions of each patient's or resident's medical record

KARDEX The Kardex card provides a one-page summary of the patient's or resident's condition and care needs. Members of the health care team can check the Kardex card instead of searching through the entire record every time they need information about the person's status and care plan.

Putting it all together!

- Reporting and recording are two methods of communication used by the health care team to make sure that everyone involved in the care of a patient or resident has current, reliable information about that person. Reporting is the spoken exchange of information between members of the health care team. Recording is the written exchange of information between members of the health care team.

- Observations may be subjective or objective. Observations are reported, recorded, or both. Observations about a change in a person's condition must be reported to the nurse immediately.

- As the member of the health care team with the most opportunity to interact with the patients or residents, you will be in a unique position to observe changes in your patients' or residents' physical or emotional status and report these observations to the nurse.

Guidelines Box 4-1   Guidelines for Recording

What you do	Why you do it
Write legibly, using dark blue or black ink, according to facility policy.	*It is important to write legibly to avoid miscommunication. A pen is used instead of a pencil because pencil can be erased, allowing someone to change the person's medical record. Dark blue and black ink reproduce best when a document is photocopied.*
Always sign or initial your entry, according to facility policy.	*By signing or initialing your entry, you indicate that you are the person who needs to be consulted if further clarification of the information you have entered is necessary. In addition, signing or initialing your entry indicates that you accept legal responsibility for what you have written.*
Only record observations that you have made, or care that you have given. Do not make entries for another person.	*By making an entry in a medical record, you accept legal responsibility for that entry. Therefore, it is best to record only information that you, personally, can vouch for.*
Date and time your entries correctly (see below).	*The date and time that actions occurred or observations were made are extremely important elements of the medical record, which is a legal account of care provided.*
Check the patient's or resident's name on the medical record and on the form where you are recording.	*By verifying the patient's or resident's identification information, you will ensure that you are recording the person's information in the correct medical record.*
Use appropriate medical terminology and facility-approved abbreviations when recording.	*Using correct terminology and abbreviations will prevent others from having to second-guess your meaning.*
Do not record care as given or procedures as performed before you have provided the care or performed the procedure. Only document after the fact.	*You may become distracted or involved in another situation that prevents you from carrying out the duties you have already charted. If you record duties as "completed" in the medical record, but then do not actually complete these duties, you will have committed fraud.*
Record information in a timely manner. If you must wait to record something, keep notes about your observations and care so that the information you record in the medical record will be accurate.	*If you wait until the end of your shift to record, you may forget important information.*
If you make an error, do not erase, use correction fluid to cover, or scribble through the mistaken entry. Simply draw a line through the mistake and initial it according to facility policy.	*Striking through an error is the only legal way to indicate a change in the medical record. Erasing or using correction fluid to correct an error could be seen as an attempt to hide or change existing information.*

(Continued)

Guidelines Box 4-1 Guidelines for Recording (Continued)

What you do	Why you do it
Remember that in a liability situation, care not recorded was care not provided.	*Proper and conscientious recording of patient or resident information protects the patient or resident, your employer, and you.*
If your facility uses computerized recording, never give anyone else your password or leave the computer active after you have used it.	*If you fail to log off after using the computer, the information on the screen may be accessible to people who are not authorized to have access to it. Additionally, if you fail to log off when you are finished with the computer, someone else could enter information under your password, and it will appear that you have entered it.*

How to Record Time

Most facilities use the 24-hour time clock ("military time") to record the time in a person's medical record. With the 24-hour time clock, it is not necessary to note whether the time is in the morning (A.M.) or evening (P.M.) because each hour has its own specific number.

When time is stated according to the 24-hour time clock, the first two numbers indicate the hour and the last two numbers indicate the minute.

On the 24-hour time clock, the hours from 1:00 A.M. to 12:00 P.M. (noon) are the same as on a regular clock. To indicate a time between 1:00 P.M. and 12:00 A.M. (midnight), add "12" to the time on the regular clock.

Examples are as follows:

Regular Clock Time	24-Hour Time
2:00 A.M.	0200
2:00 P.M.	1400
2:24 A.M.	0224
2:24 P.M.	1424

Regular Clock Time	24-Hour Time
1:00 A.M.	0100
2:00 A.M.	0200
3:00 A.M.	0300
4:00 A.M.	0400
5:00 A.M.	0500
6:00 A.M.	0600
7:00 A.M.	0700
8:00 A.M.	0800
9:00 A.M.	0900
10:00 A.M.	1000
11:00 A.M.	1100
12:00 P.M. (noon)	1200
1:00 P.M.	1300
2:00 P.M.	1400
3:00 P.M.	1500
4:00 P.M.	1600
5:00 P.M.	1700
6:00 P.M.	1800
7:00 P.M.	1900
8:00 P.M.	2000
9:00 P.M.	2100
10:00 P.M.	2200
11:00 P.M.	2300
12:00 A.M. (midnight)	2400

What did you learn?

Multiple Choice

Select the single best answer for each of the following questions.

1. Which one of the following is an open-ended question?
   a. "Are you Mrs. Brown?"
   b. "Mr. Jones, when you were growing up, what was your favorite meal?"
   c. "Are you feeling okay, Mrs. Smith?"
   d. "It's beautiful outside today, Mrs. Murphy! Do you want to go for a walk?"

2. Which one of the following is an example of positive body language?
   a. Nodding encouragingly as someone speaks
   b. Crossing your arms across your chest
   c. Tapping your feet or fingers
   d. Rolling your eyes

3. An example of an action that blocks effective communication is:
   a. Interrupting
   b. Not listening carefully
   c. Being judgmental
   d. All of the above

4. Which one of the following is an example of objective data?
   a. "Mr. Wohl says that his back hurts when he coughs."
   b. "Ms. O'Connell's urine is cloudy, and has a strong odor."
   c. "Mr. McAndrews is complaining of a headache."
   d. "The resident in room 201B is complaining of a stomachache."

5. Which one of the following is an example of nonverbal communication?
   a. Using sign language to communicate with a deaf person
   b. Recording vital sign measurements in a patient's or resident's chart
   c. Gently touching a patient or resident on the shoulder to reassure her
   d. Making a telephone call

6. What usually forms the basis for subjective data?
   a. A symptom or a patient or resident complaint
   b. A measurement
   c. A doctor's order
   d. All of the above

7. Michael is taking care of Miss Jordan, who has a hearing loss. Miss Jordan is wearing her hearing aid, but it does not seem to be working. What should Michael do first?
   a. He should raise his voice.
   b. He should make sure that the hearing aid is turned on and that the volume is high enough.
   c. He should remove the hearing aid and replace its batteries.
   d. He should report the problem to the nurse immediately.

8. With regard to telephone communication, nursing assistants are responsible for all of the following except:
   a. Writing down the caller's name and telephone number if the person the caller wants to speak to is not available, and delivering this message to the intended recipient
   b. Answering the telephone promptly, with a pleasant greeting
   c. Taking down doctor's orders if the nurse is not available and a doctor calls
   d. Identifying themselves to the caller by name and title, per facility policy

9. When recording information in a person's medical chart, what should you remember to do?
   a. Use pencil so that errors can be corrected neatly
   b. Sign or initial and date and time your entry, per facility policy
   c. Update all of your patients' or residents' charts at one time at the end of each shift
   d. All of the above

10. What is it called when people have differences and they are unable to come to an agreement?
    a. Communication
    b. Conflict
    c. Culture
    d. Personality difference
11. Mr. Campi, one of your elderly residents, is very hard of hearing. What should you remember when you are talking to Mr. Campi?
    a. You should sit or stand so that Mr. Campi has a clear view of your face, and you should avoid chewing gum or speaking quickly.
    b. If you think that Mr. Campi has not completely understood what you are saying, you should demand that he repeat it back to you so that you can correct his mistakes.
    c. If you do not understand what Mr. Campi has said, you should just let it pass. Letting him know that you did not understand might embarrass or frustrate him.
    d. There is no point in talking to Mr. Campi. He cannot hear you anyway. It is better to just write everything down.

Matching

Match each form typically found in a medical record with its description.

_____ 1. Admission sheet

_____ 2. Narrative nurse's notes

_____ 3. Medical history

_____ 4. Physician's order sheet

_____ 5. Graphic sheet

a. Used to document the person's complaints and the actions that were taken by the nursing team in response to them
b. Used to record routine data, such as vital signs, frequency of urination and bowel movements, and food and fluid intake
c. Used to order diagnostic tests and treatments and to specify dietary orders or activity status
d. Lists a person's previous surgeries and medical conditions, current medications, allergies, and current medical diagnosis
e. Contains standard information about the patient or resident, such as his or her name and address

STOP Stop and Think!

Juanita is assigned to care for Mr. Thompson today. Juanita has taken care of Mr. Thompson before, and he is not one of her favorite residents. It seems like he is always unhappy about something. As expected, the moment Juanita walks into his room, Mr. Thompson begins to complain—his children have left him here to die! His grandchildren expect him to remember their birthdays (and send money), but they never remember his! The food in this place is terrible! Juanita is focused on getting Mr. Thompson out of bed, washed, and ready for breakfast. While Juanita is busy getting the bathroom ready and collecting linens, Mr. Thompson starts to complain that his chest feels "tight," and he "can hardly breathe." Assuming that this is just another item in Mr. Thompson's long list of complaints, Juanita continues with what she was doing. If you were Juanita, would you have handled this situation differently? If so, how? If not, why not? What blocks to effective communication do you see here?

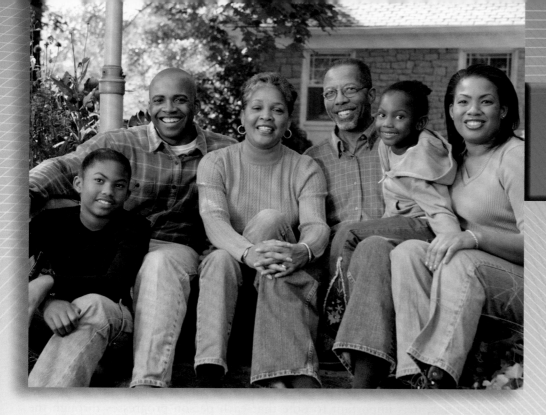

CHAPTER 5

Throughout the course of our lives, we pass through a series of stages. Here, members from the same family represent the stages of school age, adolescence, young adulthood, and middle adulthood.
(©Jupiter Images)

Those We Care For

As you are probably beginning to realize, there is much more to being a nursing assistant than blood pressures and bedpans. Those in need of health care services are not merely defined by their illnesses and disabilities. First and foremost, patients, residents, and clients are *people*. In this chapter, we will take a closer look at some of the things that all people have in common, as well as some of the things that make us different.

GROWTH AND DEVELOPMENT

What will you learn?

When you are finished with this section, you will be able to:

1. List and briefly describe the stages of human growth and development.
2. Define the words growth, development, and tasks.

Growth ■■■ changes that occur physically as a person passes through life

Development ■■■ changes that occur psychologically or socially as a person passes through life

Tasks ■■■ growth and development milestones that must be completed before a person can move on to the next stage of growth and development

Throughout our lives, we are constantly changing, from the moment our life begins until the moment it ends. This process of change is called growth and development. Growth is shown by changes in height and weight and by physical changes in the body's organ systems. Development is shown by changes in a person's behavior and way of thinking.

The process of growth and development is divided into stages of normal progression (Table 5-1). Although the stages of growth and development can be generalized by age, it is important to note that each person progresses through the stages at his or her own pace. A person cannot progress to the next stage without successfully completing the tasks associated with the stage he or she is currently in. With young children and teenagers, it is quite common to see some overlap in the stages. This is because growth and development occur unevenly or in spurts, with one part occurring faster than the other.

TABLE 5-1		**Stages of Growth and Development**		
	NAME OF STAGE	**APPROXIMATE AGE**	**MAJOR GROWTH TASKS**	**MAJOR DEVELOPMENT TASKS**
	Infancy	Birth to 1 year	New tasks are accomplished on a weekly and monthly basis; by his first birthday, an infant will typically weigh three times what he did when he was born, and he will have progressed from a totally helpless newborn to a child learning how to walk and feed himself	The infant begins to smile, laugh, recognize parents and siblings, and say simple words

TABLE 5-1		Stages of Growth and Development *(Continued)*		
	NAME OF STAGE	**APPROXIMATE AGE**	**MAJOR GROWTH TASKS**	**MAJOR DEVELOPMENT TASKS**
	Toddlerhood	1 to 3 years	Growth of the muscular and nervous systems allows the toddler to become quite active Toilet training begins as control over bladder and bowel function becomes physically possible	The toddler is able to express himself in short, complete sentences and becomes quite expressive of his emotions
	Preschool	3 to 5 years	Physical coordination continues to improve, allowing the preschooler to dress himself and tie his own shoes Toileting becomes more independent	The preschooler likes to play with other children and uses his active imagination to create detailed play stories and scenes Curiosity about the differences between boys and girls develops
	School age	5 to 12 years	Several major growth spurts lead to increases in both height and weight As fine motor skills develop, the ability to write and draw improves	Play usually involves groups of same-sex friends Logical thinking patterns develop, and the school-age child is able to incorporate other people's perspectives into her own thinking
	Adolescence	12 to 20 years	Secondary sex characteristics develop and reproductive organs begin to function (puberty occurs)	The adolescent is likely to question authority Many adolescents take jobs, learn to drive, and begin to make plans for the future

(Continued)

TABLE 5-1		Stages of Growth and Development *(Continued)*		
	NAME OF STAGE	APPROXIMATE AGE	MAJOR GROWTH TASKS	MAJOR DEVELOPMENT TASKS
	Young adulthood	20 to 40 years	Physical changes during this stage are usually minor, with the exception of pregnancy in women	The young adult focuses on completing his education, starting a career, and possibly, finding a life partner
	Middle adulthood	40 to 65 years	Early signs of aging, such as wrinkles or a few gray hairs, may start to appear Although good health is usually still enjoyed, some chronic illnesses, such as hypertension and diabetes, may be diagnosed during this stage Menopause occurs in women	Many middle adults have raised their families and now have more time to reconnect as a couple and pursue their own interests and hobbies; however, many middle adults find themselves caring for their own children as well as their aging parents Many people become grandparents during this stage
	Later adulthood	65 to 75 years	Physical signs of aging become more obvious, and the development of chronic illnesses becomes more common Strength diminishes, as do many senses, such as hearing and sight	Retirement gives the person an opportunity to travel and pursue hobbies Many people must cope with the death of a friend or a spouse
	Older adulthood	75 years +	Chronic illnesses may become more severe. Falls resulting in broken bones are common. The older adult may need assistance with routine activities, such as eating, bathing, and toileting	Many older adults enjoy sharing the wisdom of their years with younger people Although some older adults continue to be healthy and independent, many must adjust to failing health and a growing dependency on others A primary task during this stage is preparing for one's own death

Putting it all together!

- The process of growth and development is divided into stages of normal progression: infancy, toddlerhood, preschool, school age, adolescence, young adulthood, middle adulthood, later adulthood, and older adulthood.

- As a person moves through life, the growth and development changes that occur affect the type of care the person needs and the way we communicate with him or her. Becoming familiar with the various stages of growth and development will help you to become a better caregiver.

BASIC HUMAN NEEDS

What will you learn?

When you have finished with this section, you will be able to:

1. Draw Maslow's hierarchy of human needs and explain each level.

2. Describe ways that a nursing assistant helps patients and residents to meet their needs.

3. Define the word needs.

The primary focus of health care is to help provide for patients' or residents' physical and emotional **needs**. Abraham Maslow (1908–1970), an American psychologist, defined what he thought to be the basic human needs, and then arranged them in a pyramid to show that some needs are more basic than other needs (Fig. 5-1). Maslow's pyramid, called *Maslow's hierarchy of human needs*, reflects Maslow's belief that the more basic, lower-level needs must be met before the higher-level needs can be met. Many people can meet their needs with little or no outside help. But people who are ill, injured, or disabled must rely on the health care team to make sure that their needs are met.

Need ■■■ something that is essential for a person's physical and mental health

Physiologic needs

At the most basic level, we need oxygen, water, food, sleep, exercise, and shelter to survive (see Fig. 5-1). We also need the ability to remove waste products from our bodies. Meeting these physiologic, or physical, needs is of the highest priority because unless these needs are met, we will die. Assisting with meals, toileting, and ambulating and providing a relaxing environment in which to sleep are just some of the many ways you will help people to meet their most basic needs.

Safety and security needs

As a nursing assistant, you will follow many policies and procedures that are designed to keep your patients or residents safe, such as making sure that a resident who needs a walker to walk always has the walker nearby (see Fig. 5-1). Safety and security needs are both physical and emotional. When you help your patients

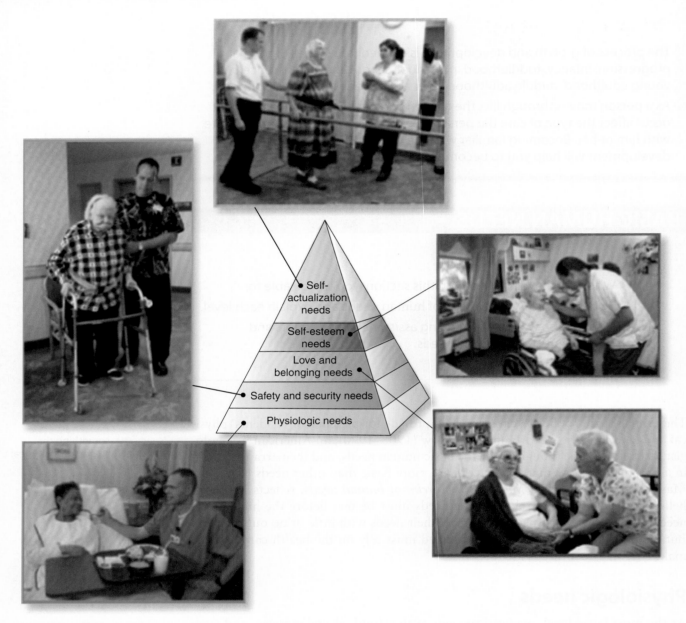

FIGURE ▪ 5-1

Maslow's pyramid. Basic needs (the needs at the bottom of the pyramid) must be met before more complex needs (the ones toward the top of the pyramid) can be met. Patients and residents who are not able to meet their needs on their own rely on members of the health care team to recognize and help meet these needs for them.

or residents to *be* safe, they also *feel* safe. They are able to relax and trust that you will take good care of them.

Love and belonging needs

All people need to feel loved, accepted, and appreciated by others. We need to feel that we are part of an accepting group. People meet this need for one another by showing affection and forming close (intimate) relationships. When our love and belonging need is unmet, feelings of loneliness and isolation develop. Being a patient or a resident in a health care facility can cause a person to feel isolated, unlovable, and unappreciated. Patients and residents often feel that they have become a medical condition instead of a person. By taking an interest in the person and showing respect for the person's specific likes and dislikes, you can help to meet that person's love and belonging needs. A smile, a kind word, or a gentle touch can go a long way toward making someone feel loved, appreciated, and like he or she "belongs" (see Fig. 5-1).

Self-esteem needs

Self-esteem is influenced by how people think of themselves and how they think others think of them. Everyone wants to be respected and thought well of by others. Many things can affect the self-esteem of a person who is receiving health care, such as:

- Having to wear a hospital gown
- Having surgery that might cause the person's appearance to change
- Having to depend on others for something one used to be able to do for oneself

Nursing assistants help to preserve their patients' and residents' self-esteem by providing for privacy when it is necessary to expose someone's body, by allowing people to wear their own clothing whenever possible, and by assisting people with basic grooming (see Fig. 5-1).

Self-actualization needs

The highest level on the hierarchy of needs is self-actualization. To achieve self-actualization, a person must reach his or her fullest potential. Most of us try throughout life to meet this need because we are constantly setting new goals for ourselves. As a nursing assistant, you will have the chance to help the people you care for achieve self-actualization by helping them to set small, realistic goals for a positive outcome. For example, when you encourage a person who has had a stroke to practice exercises learned in physical therapy, you are helping that person to get one step closer to his or her goal of being able to be independent again (see Fig.5-1).

The needs of the people you care for will change as their conditions get better or worse. By helping people to meet their most basic needs first, you will help them to meet their higher-level needs. For example, it is difficult to work on a person's self-esteem if he is struggling to breathe! Recognizing needs that people have difficulty meeting on their own and helping them to meet these needs is one of the most valuable contributions you will make as a nursing assistant.

Putting it all together!

- People in health care settings have many different physical and emotional needs. Basic needs must be met before higher-level needs can be met.
- As a nursing assistant, you will help your patients or residents to meet their physiologic needs, their safety and security needs, their love and belonging needs, their self-esteem needs, and their self-actualization needs.

HUMAN SEXUALITY AND INTIMACY

What will you learn?

When you have finished with this section, you will be able to:

1. Understand the difference between sex and sexuality.

2. Discuss ways in which nursing assistants help patients and residents to fulfill their need to be thought of as sexual beings and engage in intimate relationships with others.

3. Define the words sexuality, intimacy, sex, and masturbation.

Sexuality ▪▪▪ how a person perceives his or her maleness or femaleness

Intimacy ▪▪▪ a feeling of emotional closeness to another human being

Sex ▪▪▪ the physical activity one engages in to obtain sexual pleasure and reproduce

Sexuality and intimacy are basic human needs, common to all people, young and old. Sexuality and intimacy are not the same as sex, although a person's sexuality does influence who he or she is sexually attracted to, and sex is a part of some intimate relationships.

Sexuality is an inborn part of our personalities. A person's sexuality can be influenced by many factors, including the person's culture and religious beliefs. From birth, we are surrounded by symbols of our sexuality—little boys receive baseball mitts and miniature toolboxes "just like Dad's"; little girls receive dolls and tea sets (Fig. 5-2). We grow up being taught by our parents and peers what is appropriate behavior for a "little girl" or for a "big boy." As we progress through the developmental stages of life, we develop personal ideas and beliefs about our own sexuality.

As a nursing assistant, you will meet people whose feelings about their sexuality and the ways in which they express these feelings might be very different from your feelings about your sexuality and the way you express those feelings. You must avoid being judgmental or critical of how another person chooses to express his or her sexuality. Acceptance of another person's views does not mean that you approve of that person's beliefs and practices. It only means that you respect that person's right to make his or her own decisions.

Sexuality and intimacy are basic human needs for *all* people, including elderly people. Many elderly people are involved in, or will begin, intimate relationships,

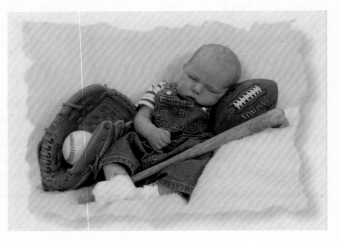

FIGURE ▪ 5-2

Society influences our ideas about our sexuality from an early age.

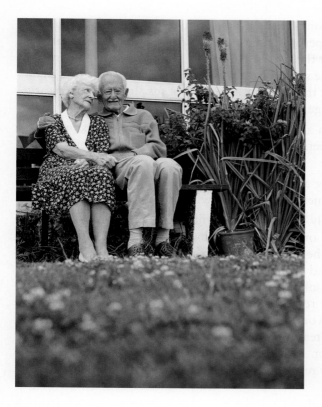

FIGURE ▪ 5-3

Sexuality and intimacy are basic human needs for everyone, young and old.

which may or may not involve sexual activity (Fig. 5-3). As we age, we still maintain an image of how we feel about our own sexuality and sexual intimacy. The desire to be clean, well groomed, and dressed attractively remains. An older person who enjoyed sexual intimacy when he or she was younger will still have those needs. Many elderly people have health problems and reduced mobility or movement of the joints that can make sexual intercourse uncomfortable. As a result, sexual intimacy does not always involve sexual intercourse. An elderly person may take great comfort in being intimate in ways such as cuddling, touching, or caressing. Masturbation, either mutual or alone, is another way that elderly people can help to meet their sexual needs.

Masturbation ▪▪▪ stimulation of the genitals for sexual pleasure or release by a means other than sexual intercourse

If you work in a long-term care facility, you must take into consideration your residents' needs for sexuality and intimacy. The Omnibus Budget Reconciliation Act (OBRA) requires that long-term care facilities allow married residents to share the same room and the same bed if their health allows. But what about unmarried residents? If two unmarried residents wish to begin a sexually intimate relationship, then this must be allowed and privacy provided. However, both residents must enter the relationship willingly. If you suspect that one resident is taking advantage of another resident, then you should report this to the nurse.

There are many ways that, as a nursing assistant, you can help patients and residents to fulfill their need to be thought of as sexual beings and to engage in intimate relationships with others:

- Avoid being judgmental.
- Help your patients and residents with rituals that make them feel either feminine or masculine, such as dressing and applying make-up, perfume, or aftershave lotion.

- Allow for privacy. If the person is in a private room, close the door and use a "do not disturb" sign as the person requests. If the person has a roommate, suggest to the roommate that the two of you take a walk or participate in another activity outside of the room. Privacy is necessary for people in intimate relationships, whether or not the relationship involves sex. It is also necessary for people who want to engage in masturbation.

- If a person is masturbating in a public room (some confused patients or residents will do this), take the person to his or her room and provide for safety and privacy.

- Always knock before entering a person's room. If you do interrupt a sexual encounter, excuse yourself quietly and say you will return later.

Some people become sexually aggressive and will behave in an unwelcome way toward you or another patient or resident. It is important for you to be able to recognize situations that could be considered sexual abuse or assault. Although it is inappropriate for you to attend to the sexual needs of your patients or residents, it is important to avoid being unkind or hateful in your response. Depending on the situation, tell the patient or resident kindly, yet firmly, that you are not going to do what he or she is asking you to do, or that he or she must not touch you in that manner. Avoid giggling or teasing the patient or resident. This will only reinforce the inappropriate behavior. If the behavior does not stop, or if the behavior is directed at another patient or resident, discuss the matter with your supervisor.

Putting it all together!

- Sexuality is how a person feels about his or her maleness or femaleness. Sexuality differs from intimacy (the need to feel close to another person) and from sex (a physical act engaged in for pleasure and reproduction). Sexuality and intimacy are basic human needs.

- As a nursing assistant, you must avoid being judgmental or critical of how another person chooses to express his or her sexuality.

- A person's feelings of sexuality and the need for intimacy continue through the older years.

- Assisting with grooming routines and providing for privacy are two ways nursing assistants help patients or residents fulfill their sexuality and intimacy needs.

CULTURE AND RELIGION

What will you learn?

When you are finished with this section, you will be able to:

1. Discuss how culture and religion can affect how a person views illness and health care.

2. Understand why it is important for health care workers to recognize their patients' and residents' cultural and religious differences.

 3. Define the words culture, race, and religion.

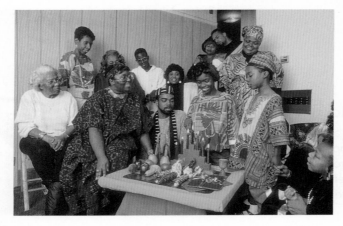

FIGURE ▪ 5-4

This African-American family is celebrating Kwanzaa, a holiday celebrated by Africans and people of African descent throughout the world. Kwanzaa, a celebration of African history and culture, with a special emphasis on family life, occurs from December 26 through January 1. Kwanzaa is a cultural holiday, not a religious one. Celebrants are united by their African heritage, not their religion.

©Lawrence Migdale.

All people have a **culture**, although everyone's culture is not the same. A culture can be shared by people of the same **race** or ethnicity, by people who live within the same geographic area or speak the same language, or by a combination of these two (Fig. 5-4).

Many different cultures are represented here in the United States. As a health care worker, it is important for you to learn as much as possible about the characteristics of other cultural or ethnic groups of people because your patients or residents will have cultural differences that may affect their preferences regarding health care. In addition, a primary goal of the nursing team is to provide for the comfort of those we care for. A person who feels that his culture is not understood or respected by the people who are caring for him will feel uncomfortable.

There are many ways in which a health care worker can accidentally be disrespectful of a patient's or resident's culture, which can lead to conflict. Sometimes, misunderstandings occur simply because a health care worker is not aware of how a certain person's culture influences his behavior. Although it is difficult to make generalizations about culture—not everyone from the same geographic region, or with the same skin tone, necessarily has the same beliefs or value system—being aware of what a patient or resident is telling you can help you to know when cultural differences need to be taken into account. Areas in which culture and health care often intersect include beliefs and practices associated with food and meals; religious beliefs and practices; and attitudes toward health, sickness, and death.

A person's **religion** is often very closely linked with his or her culture. Many people are very spiritual and find comfort and solace in prayer, reading scriptures or spiritual books, singing, and praying. You may care for patients or residents whose religious beliefs are very different from yours, but you can be certain that their beliefs are as important to them as yours are to you. Helping a person to be comforted by his spiritual beliefs does not mean that you need to share those beliefs. It only means that you respect the person's right to have those beliefs and to seek comfort from them (Fig. 5-5). If a patient or resident asks to see a spiritual

Culture ▪▪▪ the beliefs (including religious or spiritual beliefs), values, and traditions that are customary to a group of people; a view of the world that is handed down from generation to generation

Race ▪▪▪ a general characterization that describes skin color, body stature, facial features, and hair texture

Religion ▪▪▪ a person's spiritual beliefs

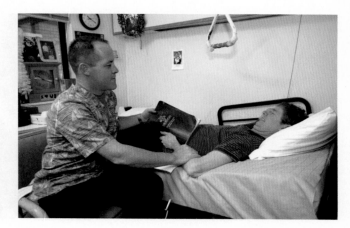

FIGURE ■ 5-5

A nursing assistant can help people to obtain comfort from their religious beliefs, even if he does not share those same beliefs.

leader or clergy member, communicate the request promptly and according to your facility's policy, and allow for privacy during the visit.

Putting it all together!

- Culture is made up of the beliefs, values, and traditions that are customary to a group of people.

- Problems can arise when people are not sensitive to, or respectful of, the cultural uniqueness of each person.

QUALITY OF LIFE

What will you learn?

When you are finished with this section, you will be able to:

1. Explain the concept of "quality of life."

2. Explain why it is important for health care workers to respect patients' and residents' decisions regarding their own quality of life.

A holistic approach to health care takes into consideration a person's emotional needs as well as his or her physical ones. To provide holistic care for your patients or residents, you must respect their decisions related to maintaining their quality of life. Quality of life has to do with getting satisfaction and comfort from the way we are living. The idea of what quality of life means is different for each person and may change as a person's situation changes.

As a nursing assistant, you will learn that a person who has diabetes must control his or her diet carefully. You will learn that a person with heart disease should stop smoking. But what if your patient or resident does not follow the recommendations of the health care team? Is a woman with diabetes a bad person if she truly loves sweets and does not want to give them up? Is a man with heart disease a bad person if he continues to smoke? What if a person refuses a treatment or surgery that may prolong his or her life? Should the health care team simply write that person off and focus only on those willing to follow medical advice?

The role of the health care team is to provide the person with all of the information she needs to make decisions concerning her own health. But then the person must make these decisions according to her personal values and sense of what is best for herself, as an individual. This is where the idea of *quality of life* comes into play. It is important to respect your patients' or residents' decisions, even if you do not agree with them.

Putting it all together!

- Quality of life has to do with getting satisfaction and comfort from the way we are living and means different things to different people.
- Allowing patients and residents to make decisions related to their quality of life is an important part of providing holistic care.

WHAT IS IT LIKE TO BE A PATIENT OR RESIDENT?

What will you learn?

When you are finished with this section, you will be able to:

1. Understand how being a patient or resident can affect how a person acts towards others.
2. Understand how it might feel to be a patient or a resident.
3. Discuss how family members may be affected by a person's illness or disability.

What is it like to be a patient? Patients feel scared and lonely. They feel sick. They are unsure about their health, now and in the future. Some patients worry about whether they will be able to return to work, and they may be concerned about how the cost of their medical care will affect their family finances. Others worry about how their illness (or its treatment) will affect their physical appearance. Patients worry about spouses, children, and pets at home and whether they are being cared for properly. They worry about the emotional effects of their illness on their family members. The hospital environment itself can be frightening and uncomfortable, full of strange noises and smells. If you were in this circumstance, how would you feel and how might this affect your behavior?

Similarly, what is it like to be a resident? Imagine what it would be like to have to move from a home you loved to a long-term care facility. You really liked your house with your cat and the shady back porch where you could sit on hot summer evenings. Now, you are not managing as well as you once did—you have fallen twice, and left the stove on a few times and forgotten about it. Even though you know that it makes sense to move to a place where there is always someone around to "take care of you," when you gave up your home, you gave up a certain amount of your independence along with it. You cannot take all of your furniture, and you must find a new home for your pet cat. You have a roommate (at your age!) and you have to eat the meals that are prepared for you, when they are served to you. Gone are the lazy summer evenings eating peaches on the porch for dinner and relaxing in the bathtub with a glass of wine. How would you feel about this loss of independence, and how might this affect your behavior?

Although some patients and residents are pleasant and grateful, others may be depressed, angry, anxious, or just mean. When you must care for a patient or resident who makes you wish you had never chosen to be a nursing assistant (and you can be certain you *will* encounter patients or residents like this), stop and think for a moment about the reasons that person may be acting out of sorts. When you look into that person's eyes, you will find your reason for choosing to be a nursing assistant . . . a person who needs you very much.

When you are providing care for a person in a health care setting, you must always remember to consider the impact that person's illness or disability can have on his or her family members and loved ones. Families, just like patients and residents, are very diverse and deal with illness and disability in many different ways. Most family members experience a sense of helplessness when someone they care for is sick. Family members may feel guilty that they are no longer able to care for an aging parent at home and now have to place him or her in a long-term care facility. These feelings may cause them to behave in ways you think are unusual. They may act angry or overly protective and it will be important that you do not take their actions personally.

If the patient or resident consents, it is very important for family members to be included in their care decisions. If the person is a resident of a long-term care facility, family members are encouraged to participate in the interdisciplinary care planning meetings and to be involved in helping to develop the resident's care plan. If you are able to allow family members to participate in the patient's or the resident's care as much as possible, it can help them to regain some sense of usefulness and control. Make sure you listen to a family member's suggestions, especially when it concerns the patient's or resident's personal preferences. In reality, you do not just provide care for the patient or resident, you also must consider the needs of the person's family.

Putting it all together!

- Adjusting to a new role—that of someone who needs the services of the health care industry—can be very difficult. Illness, disability, pain, fear, and loss of independence can cause some patients or residents to act unpleasantly toward you.

- Try to practice empathy by imagining yourself in the patient's or resident's situation. This might help you to understand behavior that is not fair or appropriate.

- It is important for you to recognize the impact that illness or disability has on a patient's or a resident's family members.

What did you learn?

Multiple Choice

Select the single best answer for each of the following questions.

1. Sally is caring for Mrs. Norville, who lives in a long-term care facility. Sally encourages Mrs. Norville to make her own decisions about what to do each day. She helps her with dressing and grooming, but lets her do as much as she can for herself. These activities help fulfill Mrs. Norville's need for:
   a. Security
   b. Shelter
   c. Spirituality
   d. Self-esteem

2. When caring for people from different cultures, you should try to:
   a. Understand and respect their special needs
   b. Encourage them to change their beliefs while in your facility
   c. Pretend that the cultural differences do not exist
   d. Avoid talking to them

3. A resident's religion forbids him from eating pork. Pork chops are being served for dinner. What should you do?
   a. Tell the resident that religious restrictions on diet do not count in times of illness
   b. Ask the nurse to call the dietary department
   c. Insist that the resident eat the pork because it contains protein, an essential nutrient
   d. Reassure the resident by telling him that the doctor ordered this diet

4. A resident in a long-term care facility may show her sexuality by doing all of the following except:
   a. Desiring sexual intercourse
   b. Engaging in public fondling
   c. Giving her granddaughter a doll for her birthday
   d. Applying make-up and scented powder before receiving a male visitor

5. Which one of the following is a basic physical need?
   a. Fear
   b. Self-actualization
   c. Self-esteem
   d. Water

6. Which one of the following is a basic social need?
   a. Food
   b. Water
   c. Air
   d. Love

Matching

Match each person with his or her stage of growth and development.

_____ 1. A 16-year-old girl going to the junior prom

_____ 2. A 42-year-old executive running his own company

_____ 3. A 2-year-old boy starting toilet training

_____ 4. A 6-month-old girl learning to sit up

_____ 5. A 92-year-old great-grandmother moving to a long-term care facility

_____ 6. A 4-year-old boy learning to tie his shoes

_____ 7. An 11-year-old Boy Scout participating in his troop's annual canned food drive

a. Infancy
b. Toddlerhood
c. Preschool
d. School age
e. Adolescence
f. Middle adulthood
g. Older adulthood

 Stop and Think!

You are caring for Mr. Spencer, whose wife passed away several years ago. When you enter his room, after knocking to announce yourself, you find Mr. Spencer being fondled by Miss Rich, another resident. You are embarrassed, as well as somewhat disgusted—you were raised to believe that sex is something that only married people engage in. What should you do?

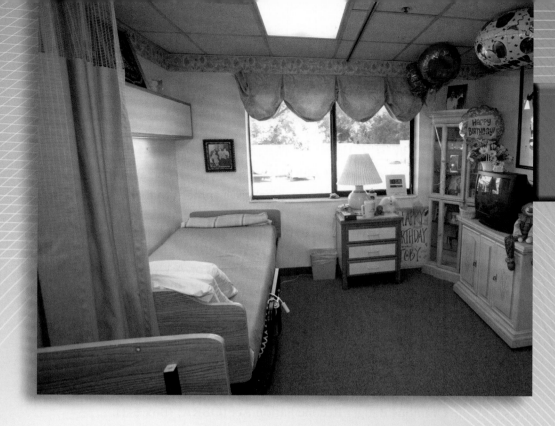

CHAPTER 6

The patient's or resident's room is considered the person's home.

The Patient's or Resident's Environment

I n this chapter, we will take a closer look at the physical environment in a health care setting and how that environment can affect a person's well-being. We will also provide an overview of the standard equipment and furniture that is typically found in a patient's or resident's room.

THE PHYSICAL ENVIRONMENT

What will you learn?

When you are finished with this section, you will be able to:

1. Discuss aspects of the physical environment that affect safety and comfort.
2. Understand your role in helping to keep the patient's or resident's environment safe and comfortable.
3. Discuss the Omnibus Budget Reconciliation Act (OBRA) regulations relating to the physical environment in long-term care facilities.

Environmental conditions, such as a facility's cleanliness, temperature, lighting, and noise level, affect safety and comfort. To ensure the safety and comfort of patients and residents, health care facilities set policies that regulate the physical environment. In long-term care facilities, standards for the resident's environment are set by the Omnibus Budget Reconciliation Act (OBRA) (Box 6-1).

Cleanliness

A health care facility must be clean and neat. Cleanliness is essential for controlling the spread of infection. In addition, one standard people use to judge the care provided by a facility is the facility's cleanliness.

Box 6-1 Aspects of the Resident's Environment Regulated by OBRA

- The size of the room.
- The lighting that must be available.
- The temperature at which the facility must be maintained (between 71°F and 81°F).
- The measures that must be taken to maintain air quality.
- The measures that must be taken to control noise.
- The types of furnishings and equipment that must be present.
- The types of modifications to the room that must be present to ensure safety (such as handrails and a call light or intercom system in the bathroom).
- The minimal amount of personal space for storage of belongings that each resident is allowed to have.
- The ability to provide privacy for each resident.
- The measures that must be taken to keep each resident's unit safe, clean, orderly, and free of obstacles where people must walk.

Members of the housekeeping (custodial) staff are responsible for routine cleaning. However, each member of the health care team also has responsibilities related to keeping the facility clean. Nursing assistants help to keep the facility clean by:

- Changing bed linens according to facility policy
- Helping patients and residents to keep their belongings neat and clean
- Wiping up spills on floors and counters promptly
- Picking up and disposing of stray pieces of trash
- Reporting problems with major housekeeping duties to the nurse

Odor control

In a health care setting, vomit (emesis), urine, feces, and wound drainage can cause unpleasant odors. Nursing assistants help to minimize odors by:

- Handling trash and soiled linens according to facility policy
- Keeping the lids on linen hampers and waste containers closed
- Emptying and cleaning emesis basins, urinals, bedside commodes, and bedpans promptly
- Using a facility-approved air freshener when appropriate
- Assisting patients and residents with routine personal care

Temperature

Most people prefer a room temperature that is between 68°F and 74°F. However, people who are ill, elderly, or relatively inactive may prefer a warmer room temperature.

Fresh air

The health care facility's ventilation system provides fresh air and keeps air circulating throughout the building. Proper ventilation is essential for carrying away unpleasant odors and preventing rooms from feeling stuffy.

Ventilation systems can create drafts (air currents), which can feel cold. Provide your patients or residents with an extra blanket, a sweater, or a lap robe as needed, and be sure to position people away from drafts created by the ventilation system.

Lighting

Good lighting is necessary for safety.

- **General lighting** provides overall light that allows people to see and move around safely. Sunlight and light from ceiling fixtures are examples of general lighting.
- **Task lighting** directs bright light toward a specific area. In a patient's or resident's room, task lighting is usually provided by a fixture mounted at the head of the bed. Task lighting helps people to see clearly when doing detailed work, such as reading or providing patient or resident care.

TELL THE NURSE !

THE PATIENT'S OR RESIDENT'S ENVIRONMENT

- A piece of equipment or furniture in the room is not working properly or has caused an injury
- A patient or resident is storing unwrapped food in a drawer or closet area
- A patient or resident, or one of his or her family members, complains that personal items are missing from the room
- You accidentally break a personal item belonging to a patient or resident
- Bathroom fixtures and floors do not appear to be properly cleaned or wastebaskets are not emptied
- There is an odor in the room that cannot be eliminated

Lighting can also affect a person's comfort level. Some people prefer a brightly lit room, while others prefer a darker room. Some people like sunlight, while others prefer light from a lamp or ceiling fixture instead. Ask each of your patients or residents what he or she prefers.

Noise control

Places that are busy tend to be noisy. In a health care facility, ringing telephones, people talking, loud television sets and radios, and equipment can all add to the noise level. Too much noise can affect the patient's or resident's ability to rest and relax. Nursing assistants help to minimize noise by:

- Answering phones promptly
- Keeping their voices down when talking to co-workers
- Reporting noisy equipment that needs to be oiled or adjusted
- Closing the person's door when the person is trying to rest
- Encouraging patients or residents to use headphones when listening to TV or music in their rooms.

Putting it all together!

- Environmental conditions, such as a room's cleanliness, temperature, noise level, and quality of light, affect how we feel.
- To enhance the comfort and safety of patients and residents, health care facilities set policies that regulate the environment within the health care facility. In long-term care facilities, these policies are designed to meet standards set by OBRA.

FURNITURE AND EQUIPMENT

What will you learn?

When you are finished with this section, you will be able to:

1. List the work areas that are common in a patient or resident unit in a health care facility.
2. Describe the standard equipment and furniture found in a person's room in a health care facility.
3. Explain how to change the height and mattress position of an adjustable bed.
4. Discuss the importance of allowing a person to have and display personal items.

5. Define the words unit, hopper, and gatches.

Unit ▪▪▪ a patient's or resident's room

The patient or resident unit is set up according to the type of care that the person needs and with the person's safety and comfort in mind.

In addition to patient and resident rooms, both acute care and long-term care facilities have similar work areas for staff use:

- The *nurses' station* serves as the central base of operations for the nursing staff. Staff members use the nurses' station to complete documentation and other paperwork, receive and make telephone calls, and monitor activity in that particular care area.
- The *medication room* is used to store medications and the supplies for administering medications.
- The *clean utility room* is used to store clean and sterile supplies, such as packaged personal care products and supplies used for medical treatments and procedures.
- The *soiled utility room* is where dirty items are handled or stored. Bins for trash and soiled linens are usually found here. This is also the room where used equipment (such as a bedside commode) is placed until it can be cleaned and disinfected. Soiled utility rooms often have a **hopper** that is used for tasks such as cleaning bedpans and rinsing clothing or linens that have been soiled with feces.
- The *nourishment room* is where snacks and beverages are stored and prepared for patients and residents.

To ensure your own safety, as well as that of your patients or residents, you must make sure that you know how to operate and adjust any furniture and equipment that is considered standard in the facility where you work.

Hopper ▪▪▪ a sink-like fixture that flushes like a toilet and is connected to a sewer line

Beds

An adjustable bed, commonly referred to as a *hospital bed*, is used in most health care settings. Adjustable beds have a crank system or electrical control device that allows the position of the bed to be adjusted. Adjustable beds also have side rails and wheels.

Manual crank system/electrical control device

Adjustable beds allow you to adjust the height of the bed and the position of the mattress. Adjusting the bed can be done by hand (manually) using a system of cranks located at the foot of the bed or it can be done using an electrical control device (Fig. 6-1). When using an electrical control device, appropriate safety precautions should be taken to avoid electrical shock (see Chapter 11). When using the crank system, remember to fold the cranks down and away under the bed after you are finished using them so that people who are walking near the foot of the bed do not bump into them.

MOVING THE BED FRAME UP AND DOWN The frame of an adjustable bed can be raised or lowered, moving the entire bed either further from or closer to the floor (Fig. 6-2). Raising the bed prevents health care workers from having to bend over so far when performing care procedures on a person who is in bed. Lowering the bed helps the patient or resident to get into or out of the bed safely.

CHANGING THE POSITION OF THE MATTRESS The mattress platform on an adjustable bed can also be positioned in a variety of ways (see Fig. 6-2). Different

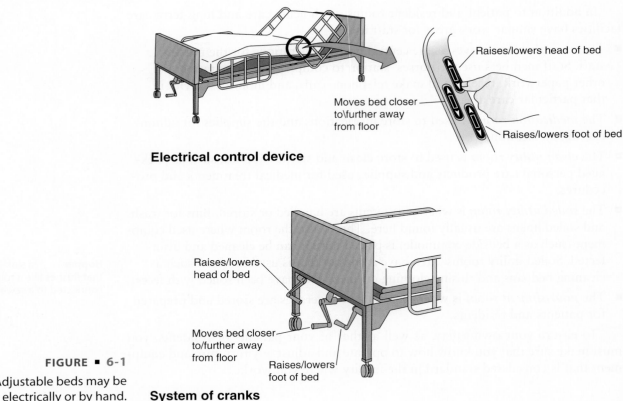

Raises/lowers head of bed

Moves bed closer to\further away from floor

Raises/lowers foot of bed

Electrical control device

Raises/lowers head of bed

Moves bed closer to/further away from floor

Raises/lowers foot of bed

System of cranks

FIGURE ▪ 6-1

Adjustable beds may be adjusted electrically or by hand.

mattress positions may be used for different activities, or the doctor may order a specific mattress position for a patient or resident.

■ Most adjustable beds permit the mattress to be "tilted" without bending the person at the waist (see Fig. 6-2). In *Trendelenburg's position*, the foot of the mattress is raised so that the person's head is lower than his or her feet. In the *reverse Trendelenburg's position*, the head of the mattress is raised so the person's head is higher than his or her feet.

Gatches ▪▪▪ the joints at the hips and knees of the mattresses of most adjustable beds that allow the mattress to "break" or bend so that the person's head can be elevated or his knees bent

■ Gatches allow the bed to bend at certain points (see Fig. 6-2). The hip gatch raises the person's upper body to a semisitting position. The knee gatch raises the person's knees to help prevent the person from sliding toward the end of the bed while sitting up.

Side rails

Adjustable beds usually have side rails that can be raised to help prevent a person from falling out of the bed. The patient or resident may also use a raised side rail as an assistive device for repositioning himself or herself in bed. Side rails are positioned according to your facility's policies and the person's individual care plan.

Wheels (casters)

Wheels make the bed easier to move from place to place, which is sometimes necessary when a person needs to be moved from one part of the facility to another without leaving his or her bed. Wheels are also useful when it is necessary to move the bed to clean underneath it. The wheels have locking devices that are used to

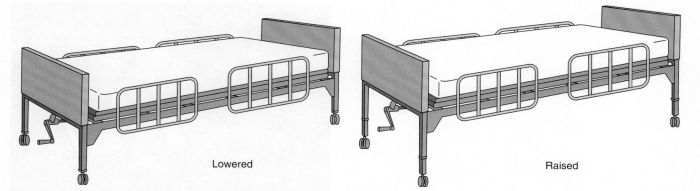

Lowered   Raised

The bed can be moved up or down in terms of distance from the floor.

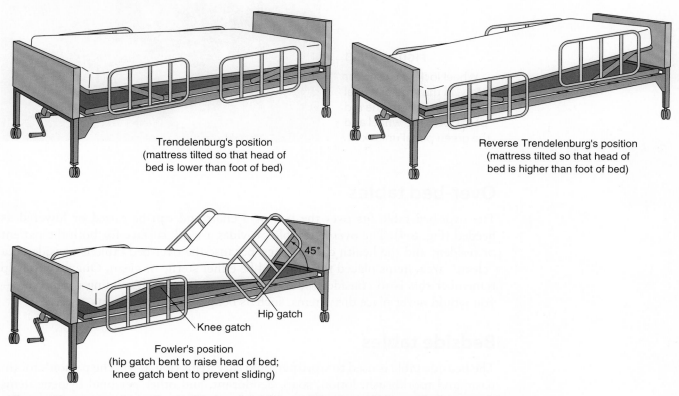

Trendelenburg's position
(mattress tilted so that head of
bed is lower than foot of bed)

Reverse Trendelenburg's position
(mattress tilted so that head of
bed is higher than foot of bed)

45°

Hip gatch

Knee gatch

Fowler's position
(hip gatch bent to raise head of bed;
knee gatch bent to prevent sliding)

The mattress can be adjusted to assist with positioning of the patient or resident.

FIGURE ■ 6-2

Adjustable beds allow you to adjust the height of the bed from the floor and the position of the mattress.

keep the bed steady and prevent it from rolling (Fig. 6-3). Always make sure the bed's wheels are locked unless you are moving it!

Chairs

A person's room should be furnished with one or two chairs that are comfortable for the person and any visitors.

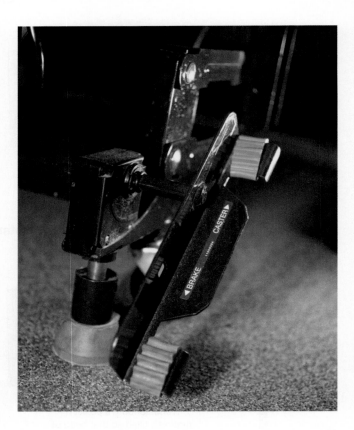

FIGURE ▪ 6-3
Wheel locks are used for safety. In the type of wheel lock shown here, the red pedal locks the wheel and the green pedal unlocks it.

Over-bed tables

The over-bed table fits over the bed or a chair and can be raised or lowered as needed (Fig. 6-4). The over-bed table provides a work surface for both the patient or resident and the health care worker. Because the over-bed table is considered a "clean" area, items placed there should be either sterile or clean. One way to help remember this is to consider the over-bed table the person's dining room table—you would never place dirty items, such as bedpans or soiled linens, there.

Bedside tables

The bedside table is used to store personal care items (Fig. 6-5). The person's toothpaste and toothbrush, lotion, soap, deodorant, and other personal hygiene items are usually stored in the top drawer. Basins, bedpans, and other care equipment are stored underneath in the lower drawers or shelves. The telephone, a flower arrangement, and other personal items may be placed on top of the bedside table.

Closets and dressers

OBRA regulations require long-term care facilities to provide each resident with enough storage space for his or her clothing and other personal items. The resident must have free access to this storage space and the items it contains. Because the resident's closet, wardrobe, or chest of drawers is considered private, personal property, you must have the person's permission to remove items from it.

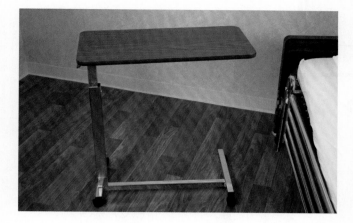

FIGURE ▪ 6-4

An over-bed table fits over a person's bed or chair to provide a work surface. The over-bed table is considered a "clean" area.

Call light and intercom systems

Call light and intercom systems are used for communication (Fig. 6-6). The call light system allows patients or residents to signal that they need help. The intercom system allows members of the health care team to communicate with patients or residents from the nurses' station. Remember, however, that a person with hearing loss may not be able to understand what you are saying over the intercom.

Answer all requests for assistance promptly. Always leave the call light control within the person's reach, whether the person is in the bed or in a chair. An unconscious or comatose person will be unable to call for help and should be checked on frequently.

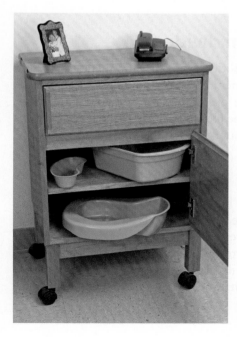

FIGURE ▪ 6-5

Personal care items are usually stored in the bedside table.

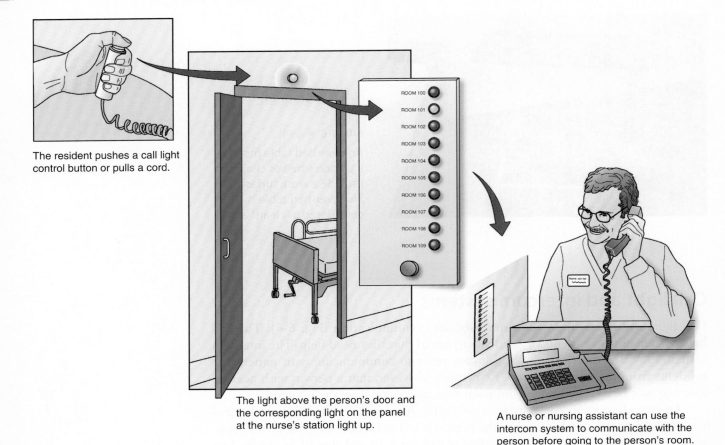

The resident pushes a call light control button or pulls a cord.

The light above the person's door and the corresponding light on the panel at the nurse's station light up.

A nurse or nursing assistant can use the intercom system to communicate with the person before going to the person's room.

FIGURE ▪ 6-6

Call light and intercom systems allow patients and residents to communicate with members of the health care team.

OBRA Privacy curtains and room dividers

OBRA regulations require long-term care facilities to use privacy curtains or room dividers to protect the privacy of each resident. The privacy curtain should be closed or a room divider used when you are providing care for your patients or residents. The door to the room should also be closed because the privacy curtains do little to keep voices and other sounds private.

Personal items

When a person enters a health care facility, he or she may bring personal items along to add a "touch of home." Usually the number and type of personal items depend on whether the stay at the health care facility is temporary or permanent. You should help your patients and residents to decorate their rooms according to their own individual taste and preference while making sure that they stay within the safety standards established by your facility and OBRA.

Putting it all together!

- In addition to patient and resident rooms, both acute and long-term care facilities have similar work areas for the staff.

- Most patient and resident units contain the same basic furniture and equipment. Making sure that you know how to use this equipment helps to keep both you and the person you are caring for safe.

- Standard furniture and equipment typically includes an adjustable bed, one or two chairs, an over-bed table, a bedside table, a closet or dresser, a call light control, and a privacy curtain or room divider.

- Adjustable beds have special features for safety and comfort. The height of an adjustable bed and the position of the mattress can be changed by hand (using a system of cranks) or using an electrical control device. Side rails are used according to the person's care plan to prevent falls. Wheels allow the bed to be moved easily but should always be locked unless the bed is being moved.

- Personal items add a "touch of home" to a person's room. Always show as much care for a person's personal items as you would for your own most treasured belongings.

> *Always respect and care for a person's personal items as if they belonged to you. Although you may consider a resident's personal things quite a bit of clutter, especially if you have to help keep them neat, just remember that each one of those items represents a piece of that person's life. When you show respect for, and take an interest in, a patient's or resident's personal belongings, you are letting the person know that you truly care for him or her.*

What did you learn?

Multiple Choice

Select the single best answer for each of the following questions.

1. How should a resident's room look?
   a. Functional and sparsely decorated
   b. Like a hospital room
   c. As home-like as possible
   d. Like a hotel room

2. You show respect to a patient or resident when you:
   a. Knock before entering his or her room
   b. Close the door and pull the privacy curtain when you are providing care
   c. Handle the person's personal belongings with care
   d. All of the above

3. Which regulations state that a resident's unit must be clean, safe, orderly, and free of obstacles in the pathway?
   a. Occupational Safety and Health Administration (OSHA) regulations
   b. Omnibus Budget Reconciliation Act (OBRA) regulations
   c. Medicare regulations
   d. Medicaid regulations

4. One of your patients has had back surgery, and the nurse asks you to position his bed so that the head of the bed is elevated. The patient's body needs to remain flat against the mattress. What position would the nurse tell you to put the patient in?
   a. Reverse Trendelenburg's position
   b. Fowler's position
   c. Prone position
   d. Trendelenburg's position

5. How can you help to control unpleasant odors in the workplace?
   a. Empty emesis basins promptly
   b. Assist your patients or residents with skin care and oral hygiene
   c. Use facility-approved air fresheners as necessary
   d. All of the above

 Stop and Think!

Mrs. Johnson is a resident at your long-term care facility. She has diabetes and knows that she needs to watch the amount of sweets that she eats. Lately, she has been having trouble controlling her blood sugar. You think that Mr. Hill, a resident who lives down the hall, has been sharing his supply of chocolates with her, and that she has the candy stored in her bedside table and closet. You share your concerns with the nurse and together you decide that you need to confront Mrs. Johnson about the candy and find it and discard it. Describe the proper way to handle this situation.

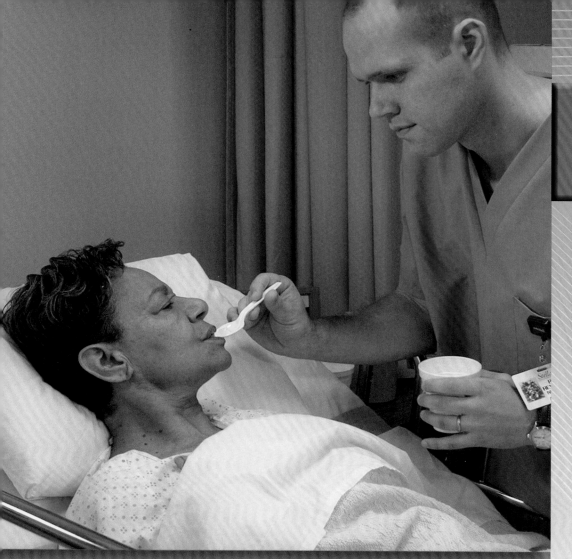

THE HUMAN BODY IN HEALTH AND DISEASE

I n this unit, we will explore how each organ system functions normally, as well as how aging, disease, and injury can affect the function of the organ system. We will also explore the measures that are taken to help the body return to its best level of functioning after injury or illness. Knowing how the body works when it is healthy helps us to understand how to help the body heal and function more effectively during illness.

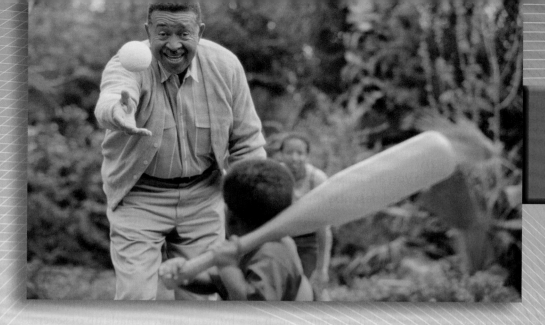

CHAPTER 7

When we are healthy, our bodies allow us to do the things we like to do.

Basic Body Structure and Function

*A*natomy is the study of what body parts look like, where they are located, how big they are, and how they connect to other body parts. *Physiology* is the study of how the body parts work. Learning about the parts of the body and how they work normally will help you to better understand how aging, disability, and disease can affect a person's abilities. This knowledge will help you to provide the type of care that each patient or resident needs from you.

HOW IS THE BODY ORGANIZED?

What will you learn?

When you are finished with this section, you will be able to:

1. List and describe the basic organizational levels of the body.
2. Define the words cell, tissue, organ, organ system, nutrients, metabolism, and homeostasis.

Cell ▪▪▪ the basic unit of life

Tissue ▪▪▪ a group of cells similar in structure and specialized to perform a specific function

Organ ▪▪▪ a group of tissues functioning together for a similar purpose

Organ system ▪▪▪ a group of organs that work together to perform a specific function for the body

Nutrients ▪▪▪ substances in food and fluids that the body uses to grow, to repair itself, and to carry out processes essential for living

Metabolism ▪▪▪ the physical and chemical changes that occur when the cells of the body change the food that we eat into energy

All living things share the same general organization (Fig. 7-1). Cells group together to form tissues. Tissues group together to form organs, and organs group together to form organ systems. A living thing, such as a human being, is made up of several organ systems, all of which work together to maintain life.

Cells

The human body is made up of millions of cells of different shapes, sizes, and functions. Each type of cell in the body has a specific duty. Our overall health depends on the ability of the cells of the body to do their jobs.

To function properly, cells need oxygen, water, nutrients, and the ability to eliminate waste products that result from metabolism. Structures inside of the cell called *organelles* help the cell to make the energy it needs to stay alive and to rid itself of waste products (Fig. 7-2). The organelles float in a jelly-like substance called *cytoplasm*. The *nucleus* of the cell is like the cell's "brain." It contains all of the information the cell needs to do its job, grow, and reproduce. A *cell membrane* surrounds the cytoplasm and gives the cell its shape.

Tissues

There are four main types of tissue in the human body:

- **Epithelial tissue** covers the outside of the body. It also lines the respiratory, digestive, and urinary systems, the inside of the blood vessels, and the inside of the chest and abdominal cavities. The purpose of epithelial tissue is protection.

FIGURE ▪ **7-1**

All living things (organisms) share the same basic levels of organization. Cells form tissues, tissues form organs, and organs form organ systems.

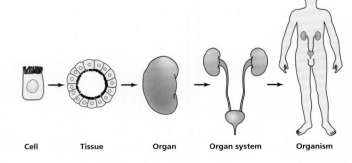

Cell   Tissue   Organ   Organ system   Organism

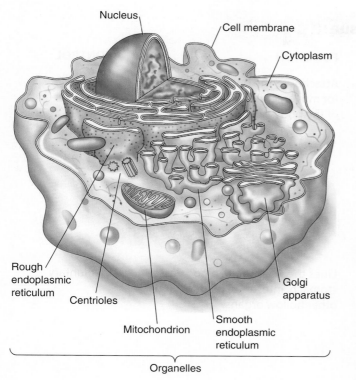

Nucleus

Cell membrane

Cytoplasm

Rough
endoplasmic
reticulum

Centrioles

Mitochondrion

Smooth
endoplasmic
reticulum

Golgi
apparatus

Organelles

FIGURE ▪ 7-2

A cell contains organelles and a nucleus, which float in a jelly-like substance called cytoplasm. A cell membrane surrounds the cytoplasm and gives the cell its shape.

- **Connective tissue** supports and forms the framework for all of the parts of the body. Examples of connective tissue are bone, cartilage, ligaments, tendons, and fatty tissues. Blood is also considered a form of connective tissue.

- **Muscle tissue** produces movement. There are three types of muscle tissue found in the body (Table 7-1). Muscle tissue is either *voluntary* (under the person's control) or *involuntary* (not under the person's control).

- **Nervous tissue** allows one part of the body to "talk" to another part. The brain, spinal cord, and nerves are made of nervous tissue.

Organs

A group of tissues working together for a similar purpose form an organ. For example, the heart is made of all four tissue types, and its main function is to pump blood throughout the body. Other examples of organs are the stomach, liver, kidneys, and lungs. An organ may have one function or it may have several.

Organ systems

For an organ system to work properly, each organ within the system must function well. All of the organ systems are constantly working together to maintain **homeostasis**. For a person to stay alive, certain conditions within the body must remain the same, within a range of normal limits. For example, the body temperature must remain within a certain range. When the external or internal

Homeostasis ▪▪▪ a state of balance

TABLE 7-1	Types of Muscle Tissue	
TYPE	**FUNCTION**	**CONTROL**
Skeletal muscle	Attaches to the bones and allows for movement of the various parts of the body	Voluntary
Smooth muscle	Lines the walls of the blood vessels, stomach, intestines, bladder, and other hollow organs	Involuntary
Cardiac muscle	Forms the heart; contraction and relaxation of this muscle pumps blood throughout the body	Involuntary

environment changes, the organ systems must make adjustments to make up for the change. Most of the time, you are not even aware of the adjustments your body is making to keep everything within the normal range. The body's ability to maintain balance is a sign of good health. Diseases and disorders can negatively affect the body's ability to maintain balance.

As we age, changes occur in all of our organ systems. These changes are not related to illness. Rather, they are normal changes that occur in everyone who reaches a certain age. However, in a person who has a disease or disorder, the physical effects of aging on the body can be increased.

Putting it all together!

- All living things are organized in the same way. Cells group together to form tissues. Tissues group together to form organs. Organs work together to form organ systems. Organ systems work together to keep the body alive.

- The body's organ systems work together to maintain homeostasis, or balance. The body's ability to maintain balance is a sign of good health.

- Because there is a good chance that many of the people you will be caring for will be elderly, it is important for you to know about the changes that normally occur in each body system with aging. Knowing about normal age-related changes will allow you to provide better care for your elderly patients or residents because you will be aware of their special needs.

> *Many people associate old age with poor physical health, disability, and a loss of mental function. But many things affect how we age—our genes, our outlook on life, and our overall health, for example. You may care for a 60-year-old who seems much older than he or she really is, while the 80-year-old down the hall may get around better than you do! Be sure to notice the real differences in all of the people you care for.*

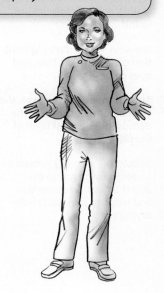

THE INTEGUMENTARY SYSTEM

What will you learn?

When you are finished with this section, you will be able to:

1. List and describe the main parts of the integumentary system.
2. Discuss the major functions of the integumentary system.
3. List the layers of the skin.
4. Describe the normal changes related to aging that occur in the integumentary system.
5. Define the words epidermis, dermis, melanin, subcutaneous tissue, and sebum.

Structure and function of the integumentary system

The integumentary system gets its name from the Latin word *integumentum*, which means "a covering." The integumentary system includes the skin and its glands, the hair, and the nails.

The integumentary system helps to maintain the body's homeostasis in three important ways:

- It protects us against germs, chemicals, and other agents that could harm the body if they were able to reach the delicate organs inside. It also helps to protect us by allowing us to sense pain, pressure, temperature, and touch.

- It helps to maintain the body's fluid balance by preventing excessive loss or absorption of water.

- It helps to regulate the temperature of the body. When we are hot, the blood vessels in the skin dilate (widen), allowing more blood to flow close to the surface of the skin. As the blood passes beneath the surface of the skin, the heat in the blood leaves the body, lowering the temperature of the blood. Similarly, when we are cold, the blood vessels in the skin constrict (become narrower), limiting the amount of blood that passes close to the surface of the body and limiting the amount of heat lost to the outside environment.

Of all the body's organ systems, the integumentary system is the most easily observed. Healthy skin is glowing and vibrant, and may range in color from very light to very dark. The condition of a person's hair and nails can also provide clues to the person's overall health.

Skin

Epidermis ▪▪▪ the outer layer of the skin

Dermis ▪▪▪ the deepest layer of the skin, where sensory receptors, blood vessels, nerves, glands, and hair follicles are found

Melanin ▪▪▪ a dark pigment that gives our skin, hair, and eyes color

Subcutaneous tissue ▪▪▪ the layer of fat that supports the dermis (the deepest layer of the skin)

Sebum ▪▪▪ an oily substance secreted by glands in the skin that lubricates the skin and helps to prevent it from drying out

The skin is the body's largest organ. The skin has two layers, the **epidermis** and the **dermis** (Fig. 7-3). **Melanin** in the epidermis helps to protect the skin from exposure to sunlight. The dermis consists of elastic connective tissue that allows it to stretch and move without damage. The dermis rests on a layer of fat called the **subcutaneous tissue** (see Fig. 7-3). The blood vessels and nerves that supply the skin begin in the subcutaneous tissue and extend into the dermis. Nerves, glands, and hair follicles are also found in the dermis.

Accessory structures

The accessory structures of the skin include the following:

- **Sebaceous (oil) glands.** These glands secrete **sebum**.
- **Sweat glands.** These glands produce a thin, watery liquid that helps to cool the body through the process of evaporation.
- **Hair.** The entire body (except for the soles of the feet and the palms of the hands) is covered in hair. Hair, especially that covering the scalp, helps to keep us warm. Hair around the eyes, such as the eyelashes and eyebrows, and in the lining of the nose helps to protect us from foreign materials and dust.
- **Nails.** Nails are made of special skin cells that have been hardened by a protein called *keratin*. Nails help to protect the ends of our fingers and toes.

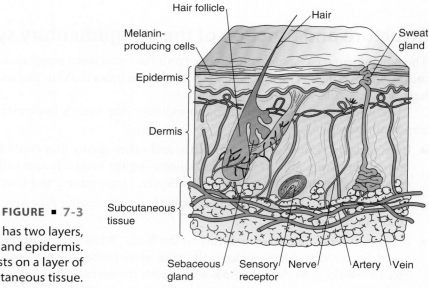

FIGURE ▪ 7-3

The skin has two layers, the dermis and epidermis. The skin rests on a layer of subcutaneous tissue.

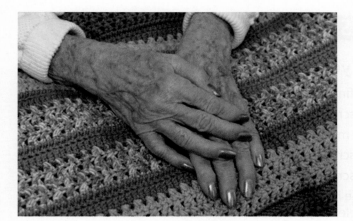

FIGURE ■ 7-4
As skin ages, it becomes more delicate and prone to injury.

The effects of aging on the integumentary system

The effects of aging on the integumentary system include the following:

- The skin becomes thin, fragile, and dry, putting the person at risk for skin injury (Fig. 7-4).
- Blood flow to the skin decreases, resulting in slower healing if injury occurs and putting the person at increased risk for infection.
- Decreased blood flow to the skin and decreased sweat production make it harder for the body to cool itself, putting the person at risk for heat-related injuries, such as heat stroke.
- The nails become thick, tough, and yellow.
- Loss of melanin causes the hair to turn gray.
- Deposits of melanin in certain areas, such as the backs of the hands and the face, lead to the formation of "age spots" (also called "liver spots").

Putting it all together!

- The integumentary system consists of the skin and its accessory structures (hair, nails, sweat glands, and sebaceous glands).
- As the body's most visible organ system, the integumentary system can provide clues to a person's overall health. As a nursing assistant, you will observe for changes in the integumentary system when you assist patients or residents with bathing, hair care, and hand and foot care.
- The integumentary system helps to maintain the body's homeostasis by offering us physical protection from germs and other harmful agents, helping us to maintain our internal fluid balance, and playing a role in temperature regulation.
- When caring for an elderly person, keep the delicate nature of older skin in mind. It is very easy to tear or scratch an older person's skin, causing it to bleed.

THE MUSCULOSKELETAL SYSTEM

What will you learn?

When you are finished with this section, you will be able to:

1. List and describe the main parts of the musculoskeletal system.
2. Discuss the main functions of the musculoskeletal system.
3. List and describe the four general types of bones.
4. List and describe the three general types of joints.
5. Describe the normal changes related to aging that occur in the musculoskeletal system.

6. Define the words skeleton, joint, cartilage, ligaments, tendons, and atrophy.

Structure and function of the musculoskeletal system

The musculoskeletal system consists of the bones, joints, and muscles. The musculoskeletal system gives structure to the body and allows us to move.

Bones

Skeleton ■■■ the framework for the body formed by the bones

The 206 bones in the human body form the skeleton (Fig. 7-5). The skeleton gives structure and shape to the body and protects key vital organs, such as the heart and the brain, from injury. The skeleton also serves as a storage site for calcium, an important mineral that keeps the bone tissue hard and is necessary for the proper functioning of skeletal and cardiac muscle. In addition, blood cells are produced in the bone marrow.

The bones of the skeleton vary in size and shape. Bones can be put in general categories according to their shape (Fig. 7-6).

Bones must be strong enough to support and protect the body, yet light enough to allow us to move. Therefore, bones have two layers. The outside of the bone is hard and solid. The inside of the bone is sponge-like and airy. Thin strands of bone form a net-like structure, and the spaces in between the thin strands of bone are filled with bone marrow. This combination of a solid, hard outside and a sponge-like inside results in bones that are strong and able to resist a great amount of force, yet lightweight.

The cells that form the bones are constantly broken down and replaced with new bone cells throughout a person's lifetime. A complex network of blood vessels supplies the bone cells with the oxygen and nutrients they need.

Joints

Joint ■■■ the area where two bones join together

Cartilage ■■■ a tough, fibrous substance found in joints and other parts of the body; in slightly movable joints, the cartilage acts as a "shock absorber"; in freely movable joints, the cartilage provides a smooth surface for the bones of the joint to move against

Joints can be classified according to the amount of movement they allow (Fig. 7-7):

■ **Fixed joints** do not permit any movement at all. The joints between the bones of the skull are examples of fixed joints.

■ **Slightly movable joints** allow for limited movement. Slightly movable joints are found between the bones in the spine and where the ribs attach to the sternum (breastbone). Cartilage fills in the space between the bones in the slightly

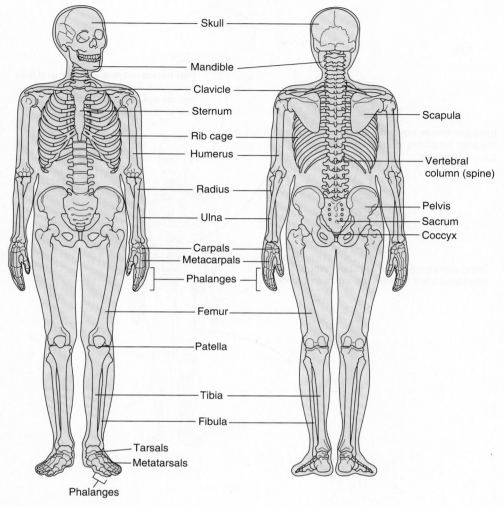

FIGURE ■ 7-5

The human skeleton contains 206 bones. Some of the major bones are labeled here.

movable joint. The cartilage permits limited movement and acts as a "shock absorber" between the bones.

■ **Freely movable joints** allow for a wide range of movement. Examples of freely movable joints include the knees, elbows, finger and toe joints, and hip joints. The ends of the bones that form the freely movable joint are covered with cartilage, which provides a smooth surface for the other bones to move against. A capsule formed of connective tissue encloses the ends of the bones, forming a *joint cavity*. The lining of the capsule secretes a thick fluid called *synovial fluid* into the joint cavity. The synovial fluid lubricates the joint, which helps the joint to move smoothly. **Ligaments** stabilize the joint. If the ligament is torn or weak, the joint may be able to move too much in any one direction.

Ligaments ■■■ very strong bands of fibrous tissue that cross over the joint capsule, attaching one bone to another and stabilizing the joint

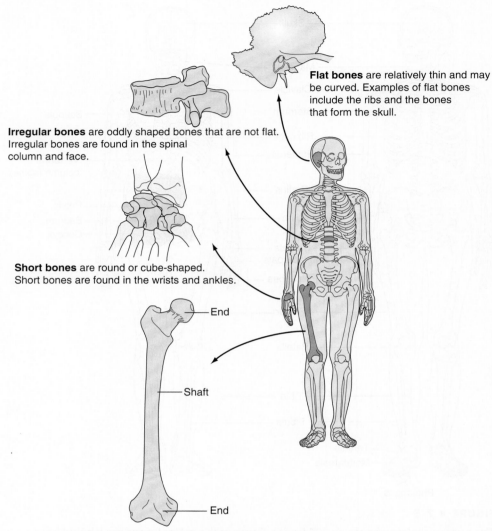

Flat bones are relatively thin and may be curved. Examples of flat bones include the ribs and the bones that form the skull.

Irregular bones are oddly shaped bones that are not flat. Irregular bones are found in the spinal column and face.

Short bones are round or cube-shaped. Short bones are found in the wrists and ankles.

End

Shaft

End

Long bones are found in the arms and the legs. Long bones have a shaft and two rounded ends.

FIGURE ■ 7-6

Bones can be classified by their shape. General types of bones include long bones, short bones, flat bones, and irregular bones.

Muscles

Skeletal muscle (see Table 7-1) is the type of muscle tissue found in the musculo-skeletal system (Fig. 7-8). Skeletal muscles vary in shape. Some are long, thick, and band-like. Others are flat or fan-like. Muscles are named according to their location, their shape, or their function.

The skeletal muscles perform three important functions for the body:

■ The skeletal muscles allow us to move. Tendons attach the skeletal muscles to the bones. In freely movable joints, each skeletal muscle attaches to the bone at two points. The two points are on opposite sides of the joint. When the muscle

Tendons ■■■ bands of connective tissue that attach the skeletal muscles to the bones

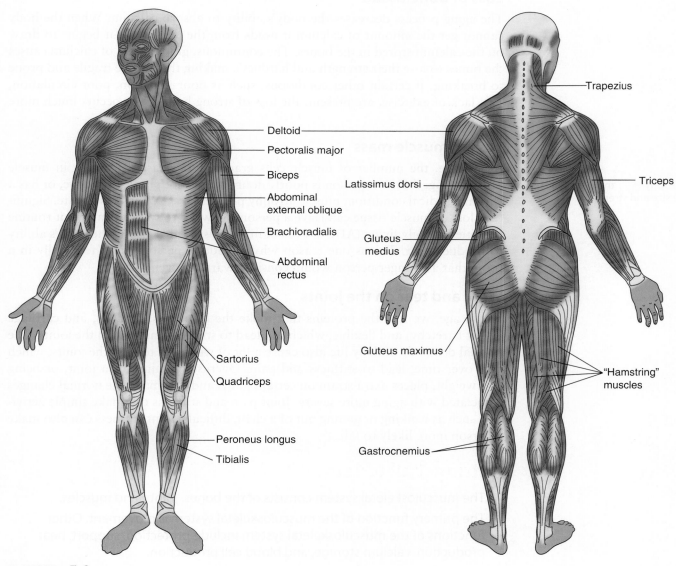

Slightly movable joint

Fixed joints

Freely movable joint

Cartilage ("shock absorber")

Muscle

Tendon

Cartilage

Ligament

FIGURE ▪ 7-7

Joints can be classified by the amount of motion they permit.

Deltoid

Pectoralis major

Biceps

Abdominal external oblique

Brachioradialis

Abdominal rectus

Sartorius

Quadriceps

Peroneus longus

Tibialis

Trapezius

Triceps

Latissimus dorsi

Gluteus medius

Gluteus maximus

"Hamstring" muscles

Gastrocnemius

FIGURE ▪ 7-8

There are more than 700 skeletal muscles in the body! Some of the more familiar ones are labeled here.

contracts, the muscle shortens and the two points are drawn closer to each other, causing the part of the body to move.

- Contraction of the skeletal muscles produces heat and helps to maintain a constant body temperature. This is why when we are cold, we may start to shiver.

- Contraction of the skeletal muscles helps us to maintain an upright posture, such as sitting or standing.

The effects of aging on the musculoskeletal system

Age-related changes affecting the musculoskeletal system are the leading cause of disability in older adults.

Loss of bone tissue

The aging process decreases the body's ability to absorb calcium. When the body cannot get the amount of calcium it needs from the diet alone, it begins to draw on the calcium stored in the bones. The continuous, gradual loss of calcium causes the bones to lose their strength and hardness, making them more fragile and prone to breaking. If certain other conditions, such as poor nutrition, poor circulation, or a lack of exercise, are present, the loss of strong bone tissue occurs much more rapidly.

Loss of muscle mass

Atrophy ▪▪▪ the loss of muscle size and strength

As we age, the number of muscle cells gradually decreases, resulting in muscle **atrophy** (Fig. 7-9). If a person is poorly nourished, is not physically active, or has a chronic medical condition, muscle atrophy progresses at a much faster rate. Significant loss of muscle tissue can leave a person too weak to walk or carry out routine activities of daily living (ADLs). Loss of muscle tissue also affects the body's ability to produce heat. This is one reason why an elderly person might feel chilly in a room that a younger person would consider warm or even hot.

Wear and tear on the joints

As we age, we lose the proteins that make the ligaments, tendons, and cartilage elastic (stretchy) and flexible, which can lead to stiffness and pain in the joints. The normal demands of daily life also cause a lot of wear and tear on the joints, which can, over time, lead to stiffness and pain. Overuse or injury of a joint, or being overweight, places extra strain on certain joints and will make the normal changes associated with aging more severe. Joint pain and stiffness can make simple activities, such as walking or getting out of a chair, difficult. Joint stiffness can also make a person more likely to fall.

Putting it all together!

- The musculoskeletal system consists of the bones, joints, and muscles.

- The primary function of the musculoskeletal system is movement. Other functions of the musculoskeletal system include protection, support, heat production, calcium storage, and blood cell production.

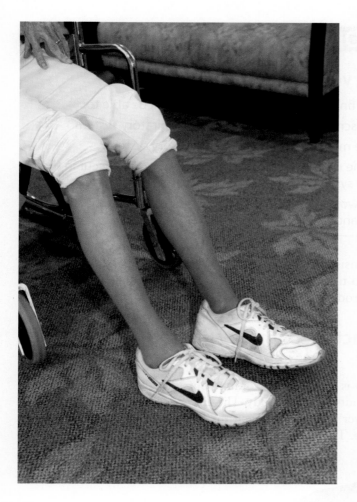

FIGURE ■ 7-9
Muscle atrophy, or loss of muscle mass, is a normal age-related change.

- Bones can be categorized by their shape. General categories include long bones, short bones, flat bones, and irregular bones.
- Joints are areas where two bones join together. Joints can be categorized by the amount of movement they permit. General categories include fixed joints, slightly movable joints, and freely movable joints.
- Skeletal muscle is the type of muscle tissue found in the musculoskeletal system. Skeletal muscle is under voluntary control. Tendons attach the skeletal muscle to the bones.
- As we age, we lose bone tissue and muscle mass, and our joints begin to show the effects of a lifetime of wear and tear. Eating a nutritious diet and exercising regularly throughout life can help to delay or decrease the effects of aging on the musculoskeletal system.

THE RESPIRATORY SYSTEM

What will you learn?

When you are finished with this section, you will be able to:

1. List and describe the main parts of the respiratory system.
2. Discuss the main functions of the respiratory system.
3. Describe the normal changes related to aging that occur in the respiratory system.
4. Define the words mucous membrane, mucus, respiration, gas exchange, and diaphragm.

The respiratory system consists of the airway and the lungs (Fig. 7-10). The respiratory system allows us to take in oxygen, which we need to live, and get rid of carbon dioxide, a waste product of cellular metabolism.

Structure and function of the respiratory system

Airway

The purpose of the airway is to move air from the outside of the body to the lungs and from the lungs to the outside of the body. The airway consists of a series of passages that become narrower as they approach the lungs. These passages are lined with a mucous membrane. The surface of the membrane is kept moist by mucus.

Mucous membrane ■■■ a special type of epithelial tissue that lines many of the organ systems in the body and is coated with mucus

Mucus ■■■ a slippery, sticky substance that is secreted by special cells and serves to keep the surfaces of mucous membranes moist

FIGURE ■ 7-10

The respiratory system consists of the lungs and a series of passages called the "airway." The structures that form the airway include the nasal cavity, pharynx, larynx, trachea, bronchi, and bronchioles.

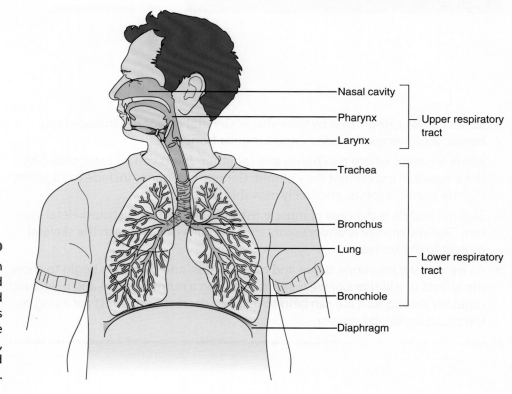

- Nasal cavity — Upper respiratory tract
- Pharynx
- Larynx
- Trachea — Lower respiratory tract
- Bronchus
- Lung
- Bronchiole
- Diaphragm

NASAL CAVITY Air enters the body through the nostrils and passes into the nasal cavity, which is lined by a mucous membrane and coarse hairs. The coarse hairs and the mucous membrane help to trap dirt, dust, and germs, preventing them from entering the delicate lungs. The warm, moist mucous membrane also heats and moistens the air. Warm, moist air is less likely than cold, dry air to damage the delicate lung tissue.

PHARYNX The pharynx is the throat. Both the nose and the mouth open into the pharynx, which means that both air and food pass through the pharynx.

LARYNX From the pharynx, air passes into the larynx. The opening of the larynx is covered by a flap of cartilage called the *epiglottis*, which snaps shut when you swallow, closing off the opening and preventing food from passing into the lower respiratory tract. In addition to serving as part of the airway, the larynx (also known as the "voice box") is the organ responsible for speech.

TRACHEA AND BRONCHI The trachea, also called the "windpipe," is the passage that carries air from the larynx down into the chest toward the lungs. "C"-shaped rings of cartilage give the trachea a ridged appearance. These cartilage rings support the trachea and keep it open. At its lower end, the trachea divides into two separate passages called the bronchi. One bronchus goes to the right lung and the other goes to the left lung.

The mucous membrane lining of the trachea and bronchi contains millions of tiny hairlike structures called *cilia*. The cilia move back and forth, moving mucus upward toward the pharynx so that it can be coughed up and removed from the respiratory tract along with any trapped particles or germs.

Lungs

The lungs are the main organs of respiration. Once inside the lungs, the bronchi divide into smaller and smaller branches called bronchioles. At the end of each bronchiole, there is a grapelike cluster of tiny air sacs called *alveoli*. Each alveolus is surrounded by a network of tiny blood vessels. Gas exchange occurs in the alveoli (Box 7-1).

The tissue of healthy lungs is very elastic and sponge-like because of all of the air-filled alveoli. The many blood vessels that surround the alveoli give healthy lung tissue its bright pink color.

The lungs are located in the chest cavity. The inside of the chest cavity is lined with a membrane called the *pleura*, which also covers the outside of the lungs. Because the lungs almost fill the chest cavity, the pleura on the outside of the lungs almost touches the pleura on the inside of the chest cavity. The pleura secretes a thin fluid that allows the lungs to slide easily against the chest cavity walls during the process of breathing.

Breathing has two phases: *inhalation* and *exhalation*. When we inhale, the diaphragm contracts, moving downward and making the chest cavity bigger. Air flows into the lungs, filling the alveoli and causing them to expand. When we exhale, the diaphragm relaxes, moving upward and pushing the air in the alveoli out of the lungs. The *intercostal muscles*, located between the ribs, also help us to breathe.

The rate and depth of breathing are controlled mainly by the brain. Special cells, called *chemoreceptors*, are located in the brain and in some of the major

Respiration ■■■ the process the body uses to obtain oxygen from the environment and remove carbon dioxide (a waste gas) from the body

Gas exchange ■■■ the transfer of oxygen into the blood, and carbon dioxide out of it

Diaphragm ■■■ the strong, dome-shaped muscle that separates the chest cavity from the abdominal cavity and assists in breathing

Box 7-1   Gas Exchange

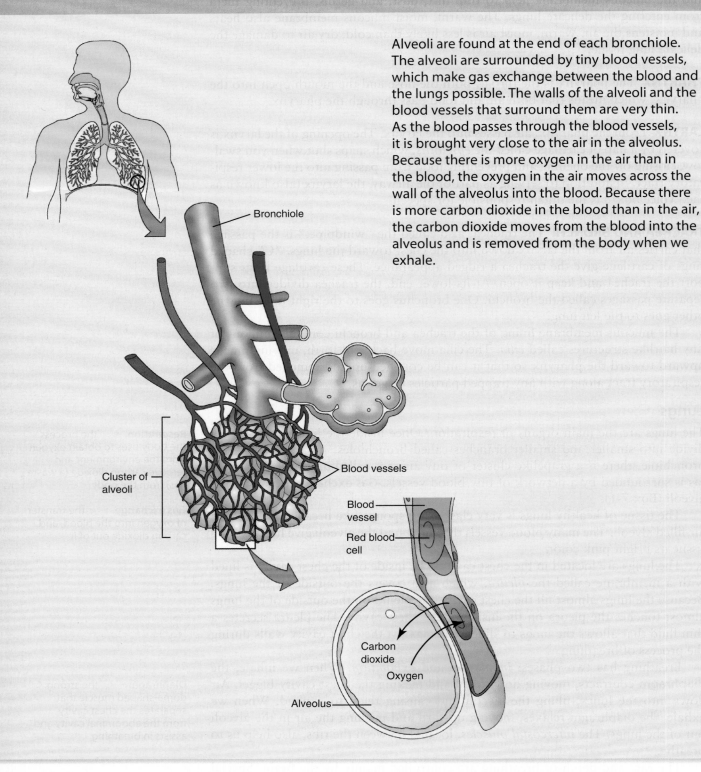

Alveoli are found at the end of each bronchiole. The alveoli are surrounded by tiny blood vessels, which make gas exchange between the blood and the lungs possible. The walls of the alveoli and the blood vessels that surround them are very thin. As the blood passes through the blood vessels, it is brought very close to the air in the alveolus. Because there is more oxygen in the air than in the blood, the oxygen in the air moves across the wall of the alveolus into the blood. Because there is more carbon dioxide in the blood than in the air, the carbon dioxide moves from the blood into the alveolus and is removed from the body when we exhale.

Bronchiole

Cluster of alveoli

Blood vessels

Blood vessel

Red blood cell

Carbon dioxide

Oxygen

Alveolus

arteries. The chemoreceptors monitor the amount of carbon dioxide and oxygen in the blood and adjust the rate and depth of breathing as necessary. Although the brain ensures that breathing occurs automatically, you also have some voluntary control over breathing (for example, when you hold your breath while swimming).

The effects of aging on the respiratory system

Exercising regularly and avoiding tobacco smoke and other pollutants help to keep the respiratory system functioning properly well into old age. However, as a person ages, there are two changes that are likely to occur to the respiratory system, even if the person is otherwise healthy:

- The lung tissue loses some of its ability to expand and bounce back.
- The diaphragm and intercostal muscles become weaker.

These changes mean that the amount of air taken in and let out with each breath is smaller.

In healthy older people who do not smoke, these changes do not usually cause any problems. Often, the person will not be aware of any change, except possibly during exercise, when the body needs more oxygen. However, when the processes of aging are combined with chronic illness, immobility, or a lifetime of exposure to toxic chemicals (such as those in pollution and tobacco smoke), the respiratory system's ability to function properly is significantly reduced. The person may have trouble breathing even at rest and be at increased risk for respiratory infections.

Putting it all together!

- The function of the respiratory system is to provide the body with oxygen and rid the body of carbon dioxide. We can live for days without food and water, but only for a few minutes without oxygen.
- Air passes through the airway on its way to and from the lungs. The structures that make up the airway are the nasal cavity, the pharynx, the larynx, the trachea, and the bronchi.
- The lungs are the main organs of respiration and gas exchange. When we inhale, the diaphragm contracts and the lungs fill with air. Once in the lungs, the oxygen in the air passes from the alveoli into the blood in the blood vessels that surround the alveoli. Each time the heart beats, the oxygen-rich blood is sent to all of the cells in the body. At the same time, carbon dioxide, a waste gas, moves from the blood into the alveoli. When we exhale, the diaphragm relaxes, pushing the air and carbon dioxide out of the lungs.
- The rate and depth of breathing are controlled mainly by the brain.
- As a person ages, the lung tissue becomes less elastic and the muscles used for breathing become weaker. These changes mean that the amount of air that is taken in with each breath is smaller. When the processes of aging are combined with chronic illness, immobility, or a lifetime exposure to toxic chemicals, the respiratory system's ability to function properly is significantly reduced.

THE CARDIOVASCULAR SYSTEM

What will you learn?

When you are finished with this section, you will be able to:

1. List and describe the main parts of the cardiovascular system.

2. Discuss the main functions of the cardiovascular system.

3. Describe the normal changes related to aging that occur in the cardiovascular system.

4. Define the words plasma, erythrocytes, hemoglobin, leukocytes, thrombocytes, circulation, cardiac cycle, systole, diastole, and varicose veins.

Plasma ▪▪▪ the liquid part of the blood

Erythrocytes ▪▪▪ red blood cells; responsible for carrying oxygen to all of the tissues of the body

Hemoglobin ▪▪▪ a protein found in red blood cells that combines with oxygen to carry it to the tissues of the body

Leukocytes ▪▪▪ white blood cells; responsible for fighting infection

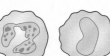

Neutrophil   Monocyte

Eosinophil   Lymphocyte

Basophil

Thrombocytes ▪▪▪ pinched-off pieces of larger cells that are found in the red bone marrow and are responsible for clotting of the blood; also *called platelets*

Structure and function of the cardiovascular system

The cardiovascular system is made up of the blood, the blood vessels, and the heart. The cardiovascular system transports oxygen, nutrients, and other important substances (for example, hormones) to the cells of the body and carries waste products away. The cardiovascular system also helps the body to fight off infection.

Blood

Blood is the life-giving fluid of our bodies. Blood consists of plasma and blood cells:

- **Plasma** is about 90% water. The other 10% is made up of substances that are dissolved in the water (such as glucose, amino acids, fats, and salts) and proteins.

- **Red blood cells** (erythrocytes) are disc-shaped cells that contain hemoglobin. When combined with oxygen, hemoglobin is bright red. As the blood circulates through the body, giving off oxygen and taking on carbon dioxide, the amount of oxygen on the hemoglobin decreases, and the blood becomes darker red in color.

- **White blood cells** (leukocytes) fight infection. There are five different types of white blood cells. Some destroy germs by surrounding them and "eating" them in a process called *phagocytosis*. Others secrete substances that cause germs to die. Still others make proteins called *antibodies*, which prevent us from getting some diseases twice.

- **Platelets** (thrombocytes) are responsible for clotting of the blood. This process, known as *hemostasis*, stops the loss of blood from the circulatory system.

Blood vessels

The blood vessels carry blood to and from all of the tissues in the body. The walls of the blood vessels have three layers: a smooth inner layer, a muscular middle layer, and a tough outer layer. The smooth muscle in the middle layer is what allows the blood vessels to constrict (narrow) or dilate (widen) according to the body's needs. Constriction slows the flow of blood, and dilation allows blood to flow more rapidly.

- **Arteries** carry blood away from the heart. As the arteries get further away from the heart, they branch into a network, becoming more and more narrow (Fig. 7-11). The smallest arteries are called *arterioles*. Arterioles send off branches called *capillaries,* which form a network in the tissues called the *capillary bed*. As blood passes through the capillary bed, the oxygen and nutrients in the blood pass into the tissues, and carbon dioxide and other waste materials from the tissues pass into the blood.

- Veins carry blood back to the heart. After the blood passes through the capillary bed, it starts its journey back to the heart by way of very tiny veins called *venules*. Venules drain into small veins, which become wider as they approach the heart (see Fig. 7-11).

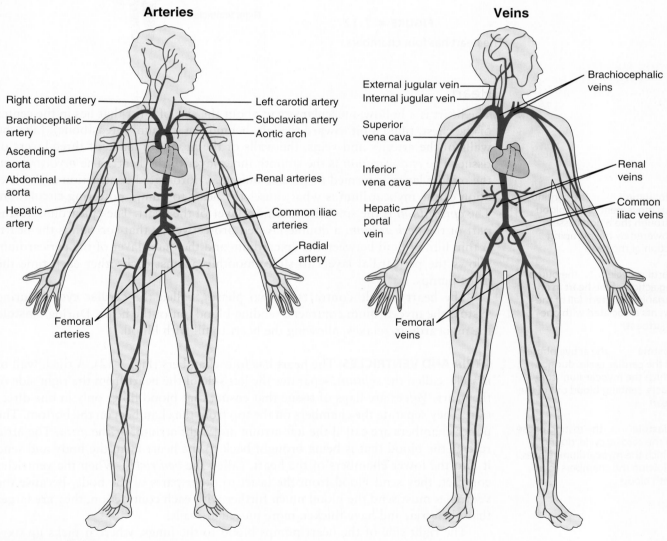

FIGURE ■ 7-11

Arteries carry blood away from the heart. Veins carry blood back to the heart. Some of the major arteries and veins are shown here.

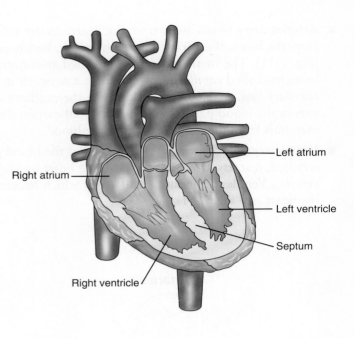

Left atrium

Right atrium

Left ventricle

Septum

Right ventricle

FIGURE ▪ 7-12

The heart has four chambers.

Heart

The heart is a hollow, muscular organ about the size of a fist that lies in the center of the chest, tilted a bit toward the left, behind the sternum (breastbone). Like the walls of the arteries and veins, the walls of the heart are made of three layers of tissue. The *endocardium* is the smooth inner layer of the heart. The *myocardium*, the middle layer, is formed of cardiac muscle. Coordinated contraction and relaxation of the myocardium is what causes the heart to pump, powering circulation. The *epicardium* is the smooth outermost layer of the heart. The epicardium forms part of the *pericardium*, a double-layered protective sac that surrounds the heart. A thin film of fluid between the epicardium and the outer layer of the pericardium allows the pericardial layers to slide smoothly against each other each time the heart pumps.

The heart muscle contracts in two phases, called the cardiac cycle. During systole the myocardium contracts, sending blood out of the heart. During diastole the myocardium relaxes, allowing the heart to fill with blood.

ATRIA AND VENTRICLES The heart has four chambers (Fig. 7-12). A thick wall of muscle, called the *septum*, separates the left side of the heart from the right side of the heart. *Valves* are flaps of tissue that ensure that blood flows only in one direction. They separate the chambers on the top from the chambers on the bottom. The upper chambers are called the left atrium and right atrium, or the *atria*. The atria receive the blood that is being brought back to the heart from the body and send it into the lower chambers of the heart, called the *ventricles*. When the ventricles contract, they send blood from the heart to other parts of the body. Because the ventricles must send the blood much further with each contraction, they are larger than the atria, and have thicker, more muscular walls.

The right side of the heart pumps blood to the lungs, where it picks up oxygen and releases carbon dioxide. This is the *pulmonary circulation*. The left side of the heart pumps the newly oxygenated blood to the body. This is the *systemic circulation*. You can learn more about the pattern of circulation in Box 7-2.

Circulation ▪▪▪ the continuous movement of the blood through the blood vessels; powered by the pumping action of the heart

Cardiac cycle ▪▪▪ the pumping action of the heart in an organized pattern (all of the events associated with one heartbeat)

Systole ▪▪▪ the active phase of the cardiac cycle, during which the myocardium contracts, sending blood out of the heart

Diastole ▪▪▪ the resting phase of the cardiac cycle, during which the myocardium relaxes, allowing the chambers to fill with blood

Box 7-2   Circulation

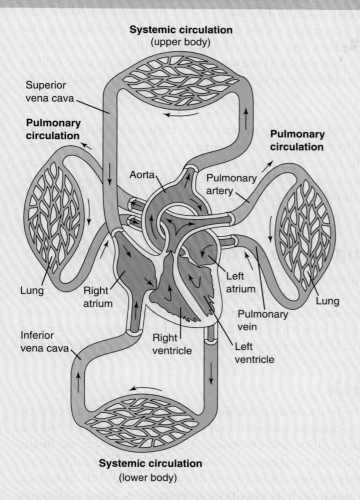

Systemic circulation
(upper body)

Superior
vena cava

**Pulmonary
circulation**

Aorta

Pulmonary
artery

**Pulmonary
circulation**

Lung

Right
atrium

Left
atrium

Lung

Inferior
vena cava

Right
ventricle

Pulmonary
vein

Left
ventricle

Systemic circulation
(lower body)

The pattern of circulation actually involves two circuits, the pulmonary circulation and the systemic circulation. Follow along on the figure. (*Red* stands for oxygen-rich blood and *blue* stands for oxygen-poor blood.)

Pulmonary circulation

- The largest veins in the body, the superior vena cava and the inferior vena cava, empty into the right atrium of the heart. The blood in these veins is returning from its journey to the tissues, so it has given up most of its oxygen and taken on a load of carbon dioxide.

- The right atrium pumps the oxygen-poor blood into the right ventricle.

- The right ventricle pumps the oxygen-poor blood into the pulmonary artery. The pulmonary artery branches into the right pulmonary artery, which goes to the right lung, and the left pulmonary artery, which goes to the left lung.

- Once in the lungs, the pulmonary arteries quickly branch into smaller arteries and arterioles to carry the oxygen-poor blood to the capillary beds surrounding the alveoli. The oxygen in the alveolus moves into the blood, and the carbon dioxide in the blood moves into the alveolus, to be exhaled from the body.

- The blood, which now contains fresh oxygen, is carried by the network of venules, then veins, to the pulmonary veins (right and left), which empty into the left atrium of the heart.

Systemic circulation

- The left atrium pumps the oxygen-rich blood into the left ventricle.

- The left ventricle pumps the oxygen-rich blood into the largest artery of the body, the aorta.

- The aorta branches very quickly into arteries that carry oxygen-rich blood to the rest of the body.

- The arteries branch into arterioles and then into capillaries, which join together to form a capillary bed. In the capillary bed, oxygen and nutrients move out of the blood and into the tissues, and carbon dioxide moves out of the tissues and into the blood.

- The blood, which now contains less oxygen, is carried by the network of venules, then veins, back to the right atrium, where the process begins again.

CONDUCTION SYSTEM The muscle cells that make up the myocardium are very specialized, so that they contract as a unit. This unified contraction is what allows the heart to work efficiently as a pump, moving blood continuously through the body. A small mass of special tissue in the heart, called the *sinoatrial node*, sets the pace for contraction by generating an electrical impulse. The electrical impulse travels through the myocardium via a special pathway called the *conduction system*. As it passes through, the electrical energy causes the cardiac muscle cells in the myocardium to contract. First the atria contract, there is a pause, and then the ventricles contract.

CORONARY CIRCULATION The tissues of the heart have their own special network of arteries and veins, just like all of the other organs in the body. The arteries and veins that supply the heart with oxygen and nutrients are called the *coronary circulation*. Coronary arteries carry oxygen-rich blood into the heart tissue. Coronary veins remove carbon dioxide and other waste products.

The effects of aging on the cardiovascular system

There are some changes to the cardiovascular system that take place simply as a result of the aging process. In a healthy older person, these changes do not have a major impact on day-to-day life. However, when the processes of aging are combined with a chronic illness or a lifetime of unhealthy habits (such as smoking, a diet high in "bad" fats, and a lack of exercise), the effect on cardiovascular function can be major.

Less efficient contraction

Changes in the tissues of the heart, such as a loss of muscle tone and a loss of elasticity, affect the ability of the heart to contract forcefully, and it takes longer for the heart to complete the cycle of filling and emptying. A healthy older person might find that he tires faster while exercising because the heart is not able to deliver oxygen and nutrients to the body in times of increased demand as efficiently as it once did. Certain medical conditions, such as obesity or hypertension, place additional strain on the heart muscle and make the effects of normal aging on the heart worse. The heart of an older person who is ill may barely be able to meet the body's needs for oxygen and nutrients when the person is at rest.

Decreased elasticity of the arteries and veins

As we age, the walls of the blood vessels lose some of their elasticity. The loss of elasticity in the muscle layer of the arteries decreases the body's ability to control blood pressure and flow because the arteries are not able to expand and "bounce back" as easily. This means that in an older person (especially one with cardiovascular disease), the arteries lose both the ability to dilate to allow for an increase in blood flow when needed and the ability to constrict back to a smaller size afterward. The "stretch" is gone from the vessel. The effects of this age-related change are especially noticeable when an older person gets up quickly after lying down. The arteries do not constrict quickly enough to maintain adequate blood flow to the brain, and the person feels dizzy or lightheaded as a result.

The loss of elasticity in the walls of the veins causes them to "stretch out," slowing the flow of blood back to the heart. Pooling of blood in the veins in the legs can cause **varicose veins**. Immobility and bed rest can make the effects of aging on the veins worse.

Decreased numbers of blood cells

The production of blood cells slows as a person ages. A decreased number of red blood cells affects the blood's ability to deliver oxygen to the tissues. A decreased number of white blood cells puts the older person at higher risk for developing infections because the body's ability to fight them off is reduced.

Varicose veins ▪▪▪ a condition that results from pooling of blood in the veins just underneath the skin, causing them to become swollen and "knotty" in appearance

Putting it all together!

- The cardiovascular system is made up of the blood, the blood vessels, and the heart.

- Blood consists of plasma and blood cells.

- The blood vessels include the arteries, which carry blood away from the heart, and the veins, which carry blood back to the heart.

- The heart, a hollow, muscular organ, pumps blood through the blood vessels. The pattern of circulation involves the pulmonary circulation and the systemic circulation. The right side of the heart (pulmonary circulation) pumps blood to the lungs to pick up oxygen. The left side of the heart (systemic circulation) pumps the oxygenated blood to the rest of the body.

- During systole, the heart contracts, sending blood out of the heart. During diastole, the heart relaxes, allowing the chambers to fill.

- As we age, changes in the tissue of the heart decrease the heart's ability to contract forcefully, which decreases the heart's ability to deliver oxygen and nutrients to the body. In a healthy older person, the effect of these age-related changes on the person's cardiovascular function may go unnoticed. But when combined with a chronic illness or a lifetime of unhealthy habits, the effect on the person's cardiovascular function can be major.

- A loss of elasticity in the muscle layer of the body's blood vessels decreases the body's ability to control blood pressure and blood flow. This is why many older people feel dizzy or lightheaded when they get up quickly after lying down.

THE NERVOUS SYSTEM

What will you learn?

When you are finished with this section, you will be able to:

1. List and describe the main parts of the nervous system.

2. Discuss the main functions of the nervous system.

3. Describe the normal changes related to aging that occur in the nervous system.

4. Define the words central nervous system, peripheral nervous system, neuron, myelin, synapse, sensory nerves, and motor nerves.

Structure and function of the nervous system

The nervous system includes the brain, spinal cord, and nerves. The nervous system controls the other organ systems. In this way, it helps to maintain the body's homeostasis by regulating what is going on inside and outside of the body and making adjustments to keep things within the range of normal. It also allows us to interact with our environment through the special senses (sight, hearing, smell, taste, and touch). The nervous system has two main divisions, the **central nervous system** and the **peripheral nervous system** (Fig. 7-13).

Nervous tissue, which forms the organs of the nervous system, is made up of a special kind of cell called a **neuron**. A neuron has dendrites, a cell body, and an axon (Fig. 7-14). *Dendrites* are short extensions from the cell body that *receive* information. The *axon* is a long extension from the cell body that sends information. The *axons* of some neurons are wrapped in **myelin**.

An electrical signal, called a *nerve impulse*, enters the neuron at the dendrites. It passes through the cell body and travels down the axon and then on to the dendrites of the next neuron in line. The axon of one neuron does not actually connect with the dendrites of the next. Instead, chemicals called *neurotransmitters* carry the nerve impulse across the **synapse**.

The central nervous system

The central nervous system is protected by three layers of connective tissue called *meninges* and the bony skull and vertebrae (Fig. 7-15). The three meninges are, from the inside out:

Central nervous system (CNS) ▪▪▪ the brain and spinal cord; responsible for receiving information, processing it, and issuing instructions

Peripheral nervous system (PNS) ▪▪▪ the nerves outside of the brain and spinal cord; receives information from the environment and carries commands from the brain and spinal cord to the other organs of the body, such as the muscles

Neuron ▪▪▪ a cell that can send and receive information

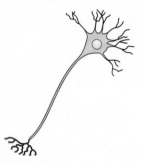

Myelin ▪▪▪ a fatty, white substance that protects the axon and helps to speed the conduction of nerve impulses along the axon

Synapse ▪▪▪ the gap between the axon of one neuron and the dendrites of the next

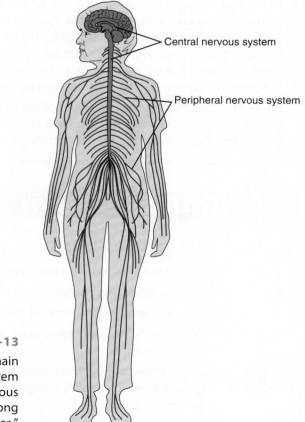

FIGURE ▪ 7-13

The nervous system has two main divisions, the central nervous system (CNS) and the peripheral nervous system (PNS). *Peripheral* means "along the edge" or "away from the center."

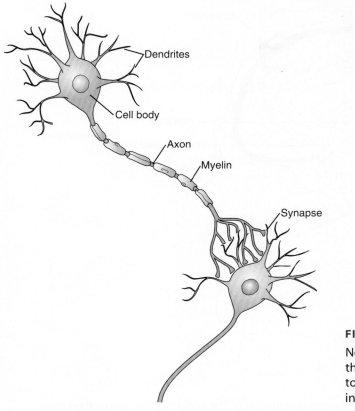

Dendrites

Cell body

Axon

Myelin

Synapse

FIGURE ■ 7-14
Neurons are special cells
that have the ability
to send and receive
information.

- The *pia mater*, a thin, delicate layer of tissue rich in blood vessels that is attached to the surface of the brain and spinal cord.
- The *arachnoid mater*, the web-like middle layer.
- The *dura mater*, a thick, tough outer layer that is attached to the inside of the skull and the vertebrae.

The space between the pia mater and the arachnoid mater contains **cerebro-spinal fluid (CSF)**.

THE BRAIN   The brain is where information is processed and instructions are issued. The brain has four parts: the cerebrum, the diencephalon, the brain stem, and the cerebellum (see Fig. 7-15).

Cerebrum   The cerebrum is the largest part of the brain, with the characteristic "folds" that we always picture when we think of a brain. The cerebrum:

- Controls the voluntary movement of muscles
- Gives meaning to information received from the eyes, ears, nose, taste buds, and sensory receptors in the skin
- Allows us to speak, remember, think, and feel emotions

A deep groove divides the cerebrum into two halves, the "left brain" and the "right brain." The right side of the brain controls the left side of the body, and vice versa. So, an injury to the tissues in the left side of the brain may result in loss of function on the right side of the body.

Cerebrospinal fluid (CSF) ■■■
a clear fluid that circulates around the brain and spinal cord and acts as a "shock absorber" to protect these structures

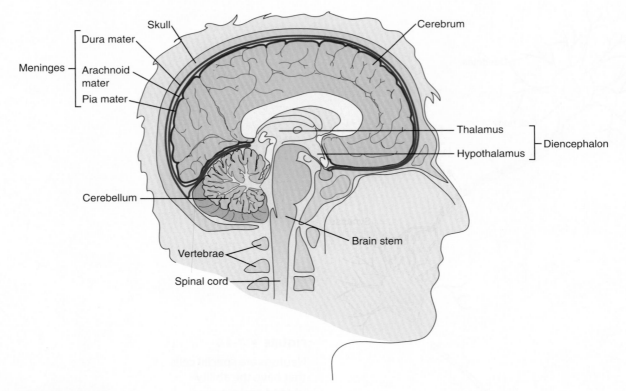

FIGURE ▪ 7-15

The brain and the spinal cord make up the central nervous system (CNS). The brain has four parts: the cerebrum, the diencephalon, the brain stem, and the cerebellum. Three layers of connective tissue, called the dura mater, the arachnoid mater, and the pia mater, help to cushion and protect the brain and spinal cord. Additional protection is provided by the bony skull and vertebrae.

Diencephalon The diencephalon is made up of the *thalamus* and the *hypothalamus*. The thalamus is responsible for sorting out the impulses that arrive via the spinal cord from other parts of the body and sending them to the correct part of the cerebrum. The hypothalamus controls body temperature, fluid balance, appetite, sleep cycles, and some of the emotions and regulates the pituitary gland.

Brain stem The brain stem connects the spinal cord to the brain. The brain stem contains the centers that control respiration, heartbeat, and blood pressure.

Cerebellum The cerebellum helps to coordinate the brain's commands to the muscles so that the muscles move smoothly and in an orderly fashion. It also plays a role in balance.

THE SPINAL CORD The spinal cord is a "cord" of nervous tissue that extends from the base of the brain downward to a point approximately even with your bellybutton. The spinal cord is the main connection between the brain and the rest of the body. The *vertebrae* (the bones that make up your spine) surround and protect the spinal cord.

The peripheral nervous system

The peripheral nervous system consists of the nerves that supply every part of the body. The nerves that form the peripheral nervous system are either sensory nerves or motor nerves. **Sensory nerves** carry information from the "outside in." **Motor nerves** carry information from the "inside out."

Thirty-one pairs of nerves, called *spinal nerves*, connect to the spinal cord. Each spinal nerve consists of one sensory nerve and one motor nerve.

Twelve pairs of nerves, called *cranial nerves*, connect directly to the brain. The cranial nerves are responsible for many of our special senses, such as sight, smell, hearing, and taste.

Sensory nerves ■■■ nerves that carry information from the internal organs and the outside world to the spinal cord and up into the brain so that the brain can analyze the information

Motor nerves ■■■ nerves that carry commands from the brain down the spinal cord and out to the muscles and organs of the body

The effects of aging on the nervous system

Slower reaction times

You may notice that some of your elderly patients or residents are not as quick to react to things as they used to be. As we age, the amount of myelin surrounding the axons decreases, reducing the speed of nerve conduction by approximately 10 percent. In addition, chemical imbalances can interfere with the ability of a nerve impulse to travel across a synapse, slowing conduction. These changes are a normal part of the aging process, and they occur gradually over time. Slowed conduction times can increase an elderly person's risk for falling and having other household accidents.

Memory changes

Memory and thought processes usually remain intact with normal aging. It may take an older person slightly longer to remember names, dates, or other information from the past, but given enough time, the person will eventually remember. Many older people experience a mild loss of memory for recent events while still having excellent long-term memory. Extreme memory loss, such as that seen in people with dementia, is not a normal age-related change.

Putting it all together!

- The nervous system receives, processes, and responds to information, helping the body to maintain a state of homeostasis.
- The nervous system is divided into the central nervous system and the peripheral nervous system. The central nervous system is made up of the brain and spinal cord. The peripheral nervous system is made up of the nerves.
- As we age, our reaction times become slower and we may experience slight memory loss.

THE SENSORY SYSTEM

What will you learn?

When you are finished with this section, you will be able to:

1. Discuss the main functions of the sensory system.
2. Describe how we sense touch, position, and pain.

3. Describe how we experience taste and smell.

4. Describe how we experience sight.

5. Describe how we experience sound.

6. Describe the normal changes related to aging that occur in the sensory system.

7. Define the words sensory receptors, cerumen, presbyopia, and presbycusis.

Structure and function of the sensory system

The sensory system is the part of the nervous system that protects us from harm and lets us experience the world that we live in. The sensory system consists of sensory receptors. The sensory receptor picks up information, called a *stimulus*, and translates it into a nerve impulse, which is then sent to the brain for interpretation via the sensory nerve. Some sensory receptors are found in the *sense organs*—the eyes, the ears, the nose, and the taste buds. Other sensory receptors are found throughout the skin, and even in the tissues of internal organs.

General sense

General sense is responsible for our sense of touch, position, and pain. The sensory receptors that are responsible for general sense are found throughout the body.

TOUCH Our sense of touch allows us to feel textures and the shapes of objects. Sensory receptors are stimulated when something comes in contact with the surface of the body and presses on them, causing them to change shape. Some areas of the body, such as the fingers and lips, have more sensory receptors than others, and are therefore more sensitive to touch.

Some of the sensory receptors in the skin allow us to sense pressure, also known as *deep touch*. The discomfort caused by prolonged pressure is what makes us shift our position when we have been sitting in one position for a long time. A person who is unable to sense pressure (for example, a person who is paralyzed) does not become uncomfortable from being in one position for a long time.

POSITION Sensory receptors found in the muscles, tendons, and joints keep the brain informed about the position of various body parts in relation to each other. For example, you can tell if your leg is bent or straight without actually looking down to check its position. These same receptors also relay information to the brain about the degree of muscle contraction, especially when the muscle is contracting against resistance (for example, when you are lifting weights). Position sense provides us with muscle tone and the ability to move our muscles in a smooth, coordinated way.

PAIN Pain tells us that we have been injured, that we have overworked a muscle group, that an organ is not working properly, or that we are ill. Free nerve endings (dendrites) in the skin and the tissues of our internal organs allow us to detect pain.

Sensory receptors ▪▪▪
specialized cells or groups of cells associated with a sensory nerve

Taste and smell

Sensory receptors on the tongue and in the nose allow us to taste and smell. These sensory receptors detect chemicals in the food we eat, the beverages we drink, and the air we breathe. The chemical signal is changed to an electrical one and carried by sensory neurons to the brain, which tells us what we are tasting or smelling.

Sight

Our eyes contain sensory receptors for vision. The eyes are protected by the bones of the skull and by the eyelashes, eyebrows, and tears. Skeletal muscles located around the eyeball allow us to move our eyes. The eyeball is made up of three layers of tissue (Fig. 7-16):

- The *sclera* is the tough outer layer. The sclera is made of connective tissue. Although most of the sclera is white, the front of the sclera, which is called the *cornea*, is clear. Light passes through the cornea to the inside of the eye.

- The *choroid* is the middle layer. This layer contains the blood vessels that supply the retina and other parts of the eye. At the front of the eye, the choroid also forms the ciliary body and the iris. The *ciliary body* is a muscular structure that attaches to the *lens*, a flexible, transparent, curved structure that adjusts to focus light rays onto the retina. The ciliary body changes the shape of the lens, allowing the eye to focus. The *iris* is the colored part of the eye. The iris is actually a round muscle with an opening in the center (the *pupil*). The iris controls the amount of light that enters the eye through the pupil.

- The *retina* is the innermost layer. The retina contains sensory receptors, called rods and cones, which turn light into nerve impulses. The nerve impulses travel through the *optic nerve* to the brain for interpretation.

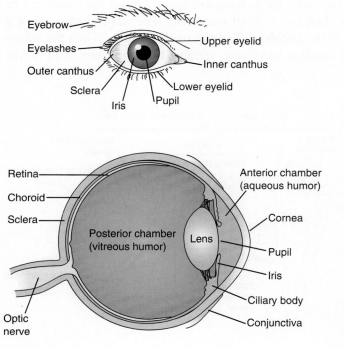

FIGURE ▪ 7-16

The eye.

The eyeball also has two fluid-filled chambers (see Fig. 7-16):

- The *anterior chamber* is located between the cornea and the lens. Special cells in the ciliary body secrete *aqueous humor*, a watery fluid that fills the anterior chamber. The aqueous humor passes through the anterior chamber and is reabsorbed back into the bloodstream.

- The *posterior chamber* is located between the lens and the retina. The posterior chamber is filled with *vitreous humor*, a jelly-like substance that gives the eyeball its shape.

Hearing and balance

The sense organ of hearing and balance is the ear (Fig. 7-17).

OUTER EAR The outer ear consists of the part of the ear that you can see (called the *pinna* or the *auricle*) plus a short canal called the *external auditory canal*. The external auditory canal is lined with small hairs and special glands that secrete cerumen. The shape of the pinna allows it to collect sound waves and direct them down the external auditory canal toward the *tympanic membrane* (*eardrum*).

MIDDLE EAR The middle ear consists of an air space containing three small bones (called *ossicles*) and the opening of the *eustachian tube*. The eustachian tube connects the middle ear to the pharynx (throat) and helps to balance the pressure in the middle ear.

The three small bones in the middle ear, called the *malleus*, the *incus*, and the *stapes*, form a tiny bridge between the tympanic membrane and the inner ear. As the sound waves travel down the external auditory canal, they cause the tympanic membrane to vibrate. The tympanic membrane vibrations are then passed to the malleus, which sends the vibrations to the incus and then to the stapes.

INNER EAR The inner ear contains the sensory receptors that make hearing and balance possible. Sensory receptors for hearing are found within the *cochlea*. The cochlea looks like a snail's shell and is filled with fluid. The stapes rests against a membrane at the opening of the cochlea called the *oval window*. When the stapes vibrates, it causes the oval window to vibrate, sending the vibrations through the

Cerumen ▪▪▪ a waxy substance that helps to protect the external auditory canal by trapping dirt and other particles; commonly referred to as "earwax"

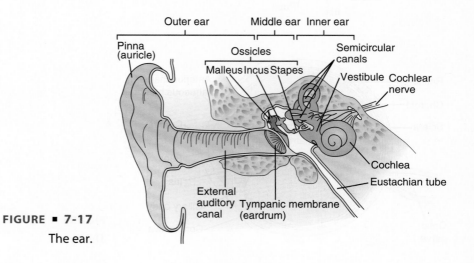

FIGURE ▪ 7-17

The ear.

fluid inside the cochlea. The moving fluid stimulates the sensory receptors inside the cochlea, which then send nerve impulses via the cochlear nerve to the brain. The brain interprets these nerve impulses as sound.

The other part of the inner ear consists of two sac-like structures called the *vestibule* and three *semicircular canals*. The vestibule and the semicircular canals, which are referred to together as the *vestibular apparatus*, help us to keep our balance. Like the cochlea, the semicircular canals are filled with fluid. When your body position changes, sensory receptors in the vestibular apparatus are stimulated. These sensory receptors then send nerve impulses via the vestibular nerve to the brain. These nerve impulses tell the brain what the body's position is relative to the ground.

The effects of aging on the sensory system

Age-related changes that affect the sensory system can put an older person at risk for harm. They may also make it more difficult for the person to communicate with others.

- **General sense.** The sense of touch becomes diminished because of the loss of sensory receptors in the skin. This can put the person at risk for accidental burns.

- **Taste and smell.** The senses of taste and smell become weaker due to a decreased number of chemoreceptors on the tongue and on the roof of the nasal cavity. This can lead to a decrease in appetite. It can also put the older person at risk for injury. For example, an older person may not be able to tell that food has spoiled and so may become ill from eating it. Similarly, he or she may not be able to detect the smell of smoke or a gas leak.

- **Sight.** Changes in the eye as a result of aging can lead to presbyopia and dry eyes. In addition, older people need more time to adjust when moving from a brightly lit area to a dim one or vice versa.

- **Hearing.** Many older people gradually develop presbycusis. A person with presbycusis has trouble telling the difference between similar-sounding high-pitched sounds like *th* and *s*, which can lead to frequent misunderstandings. Many older people with presbycusis are mistakenly labeled "confused" or "disoriented" by family members, friends, or health care workers, but in fact, they just cannot hear well. A person with presbycusis may have trouble following conversations, especially when many people are talking at once or there is a lot of background noise. As a result, the person may start to avoid social situations because he or she cannot hear well and is embarrassed to have to keep asking others to repeat themselves. Avoiding social gatherings can lead to a feeling of isolation and a decreased quality of life for the older person. When speaking with a person with presbycusis, speak slowly and use a lower tone of voice. This may make it easier for the person to understand what you are saying.

Presbyopia ■■■ age-related loss of the eye's ability to focus on objects that are close

Presbycusis ■■■ age-related hearing loss

Putting it all together!

- Our sensory system protects us from harm and lets us experience the world that we live in.

- Sensory receptors are found throughout the body and allow us to sense touch, position, and pain.

- Sensory receptors are also located in the specific sense organs: the eyes, ears, nose, and tongue.
- Age-related changes that affect the sensory system can put the older person at risk for injury and may make it harder for the person to communicate with others. Normal age-related changes include a decreased sense of taste and smell, presbyopia (an inability to focus on objects that are close), and presbycusis (age-related hearing loss).

THE ENDOCRINE SYSTEM

What will you learn?

When you are finished with this section, you will be able to:

1. Discuss the main function of the endocrine system.
2. List and describe the glands that make up the endocrine system.
3. List the hormones produced by the different glands of the endocrine system.
4. Describe the normal changes related to aging that occur in the endocrine system.

5. Define the word hormones.

Structure and function of the endocrine system

The endocrine system consists of glands throughout the body (Table 7-2). The endocrine system controls many of the body's processes, such as growth and development, reproduction, and metabolism. It does this by producing hormones, which are released into the bloodstream. The hormone travels in the blood until it reaches the specific cells that it acts on. Some hormones act on all of the body's cells, while other hormones act on only certain types of cells. Sometimes, the effects of the hormone occur over a long period of time. Other times, the effects of hormones occur more quickly. Hormones with short-term effects help the body to maintain homeostasis.

Hormones ▪▪▪ chemicals that act on cells to produce a response

Pituitary gland

The pituitary gland is connected by a stalk to the hypothalamus (part of the brain). The hypothalamus controls the pituitary gland. The pituitary gland releases hormones that affect other glands in the endocrine system. In this sense, the pituitary gland is like the "master gland." The pituitary gland has two parts, the posterior lobe and the anterior lobe (Fig. 7-18).

Thyroid gland

The thyroid gland secretes thyroxine and calcitonin:

- *Thyroxine* sets the metabolism rate for the body's cells.
- *Calcitonin* lowers the amount of calcium in the bloodstream by allowing the calcium to be stored in the bones and eliminated by the kidneys.

TABLE 7-2	The Endocrine System

GLAND	HORMONES	EFFECT ON BODY
Pineal gland	Melatonin	Regulates sleep–wake cycles
Pituitary gland	Adrenocorticotropic hormone (ACTH) Thyroid-stimulating hormone (TSH) Gonadotropins Prolactin Growth hormone Oxytocin Antidiuretic hormone (ADH)	Controls other glands in the endocrine system
Thyroid gland	Thyroxine Calcitonin	Sets the metabolism rate for the body's cells Lowers the amount of calcium in the bloodstream by allowing calcium to be deposited in the bones and eliminated by the kidneys
Parathyroid glands (behind thyroid gland)	Parathyroid hormone (PTH)	Causes calcium to be released from the bones into the bloodstream
Thymus	Thymosin	Helps infection-fighting cells mature
Adrenal glands	Epinephrine Norepinephrine Glucocorticoids Mineralocorticoids Androgens	Help manage stress, metabolize fats and proteins, regulate the level of certain minerals in the body, and produce sex hormones
Pancreas	Insulin Glucagon	Lowers blood glucose levels Raises blood glucose levels
Sex glands: Ovaries (female) Testes (male)	Sex hormones	Regulate reproduction

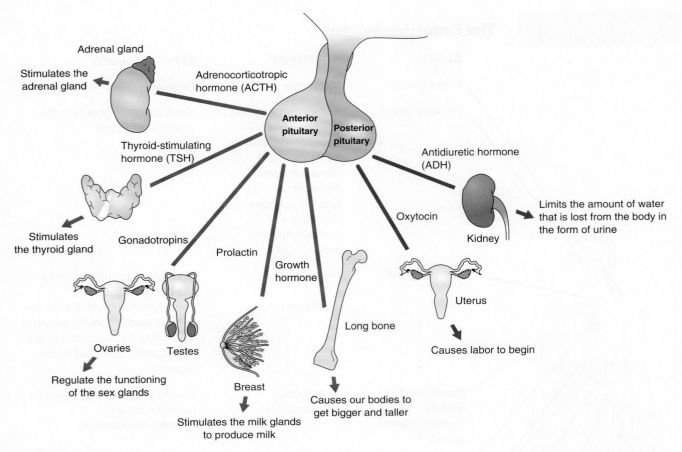

FIGURE ■ 7-18

The pituitary gland, or "master gland," releases hormones that affect other glands in the endocrine system.

Adrenal glands

The adrenal glands are located on top of the kidneys. Each adrenal gland has two parts: the *medulla*, or inner portion, and the *cortex*, or outer portion. The medulla secretes *epinephrine* (adrenaline) and *norepinephrine*, two hormones that are responsible for the "fight-or-flight" response of the body in emergency situations. The cortex secretes:

■ *Glucocorticoids*, which play a role in the metabolism of fats and proteins and help the body to maintain a reserve of glucose (sugar) that can be used in times of stress

■ *Mineralocorticoids*, which help to regulate the level of certain minerals in the body, particularly sodium and potassium

■ *Androgens*, which are changed by the body into the sex hormones *testosterone* (in men) and estradiol (in women)

Pancreas

The pancreas produces insulin and glucagon, which work together to keep the body's blood glucose levels stable:

■ *Insulin* allows glucose to be transported from the bloodstream into the individual cells, where it is used for energy. In this way, insulin lowers the blood glucose level.

- *Glucagon* raises the blood glucose level by stimulating the liver to release stored glucose into the bloodstream.

The effects of aging on the endocrine system

The normal processes of aging decrease the amount of hormones produced and slow their secretion by the glands of the endocrine system. Many of the changes that are part of aging are directly related to the smaller amounts of hormone released. For example, decreased hormone production causes women to enter menopause.

Putting it all together!

- The endocrine system is made up of glands throughout the body that produce hormones. Hormones are chemical messengers that allow the body to reproduce, grow, develop, metabolize energy, respond to stress and injury, and maintain homeostasis.

- The pituitary gland is commonly called the "master gland" because it regulates the function of the other endocrine glands throughout the body.

- The thyroid gland produces thyroxine, which helps to regulate metabolism, and calcitonin, which helps to maintain calcium levels in the bloodstream.

- The adrenal glands produce hormones that help us to deal with stress.

- The pancreas secretes insulin and glucagon, which play a role in regulating blood glucose levels.

- Many of the physical changes that are part of aging are directly related to a decrease in the amount of hormones released throughout the body.

THE DIGESTIVE SYSTEM

What will you learn?

When you are finished with this section, you will be able to:

1. List and describe the main parts of the digestive system.
2. Discuss the main functions of the digestive system.
3. Describe the normal changes related to aging that occur in the digestive system.

4. Define the words feces, peristalsis, digestion, enzymes, absorption, and constipation.

Structure and function of the digestive system

The digestive system breaks down the food we eat into nutrients, which are then absorbed into the bloodstream for use by the body's cells. The digestive system also removes unusable digested food from the body, in the form of feces.

Feces ■■■ the semi-solid waste product of digestion; stool

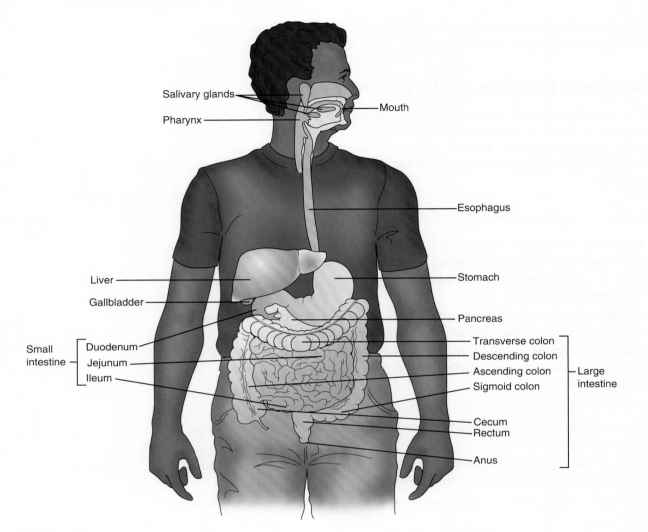

Salivary glands
Pharynx
Mouth
Esophagus
Liver
Gallbladder
Stomach
Pancreas
Small intestine — Duodenum, Jejunum, Ileum
Transverse colon
Descending colon
Ascending colon
Sigmoid colon
Large intestine
Cecum
Rectum
Anus

FIGURE ■ 7-19

The digestive system.

The digestive system is a long tube, or *tract*, consisting of the mouth, pharynx, esophagus, stomach, small intestine, and large intestine (Fig. 7-19). The walls of the "tube" are made up of four layers of tissue. The layers are basically the same throughout the digestive tract, although there is some variation from region to region. The inner layer, called the *mucosa*, secretes mucus and helps to protect us from germs and from the harsh chemicals found in stomach acid. The next layer, the *submucosa*, contains the blood vessels and nerves that supply the digestive tract. The *muscle* layer contains smooth muscle, which contracts and relaxes, allowing **peristalsis** to occur. The *serosa* is a tough outer layer of connective tissue.

In addition, several accessory organs—the teeth, salivary glands, liver, gallbladder, and pancreas—play a role in digestion but are not actually part of the digestive tract (see Fig. 7-19).

■ The *teeth* are located in the mouth and assist with chewing food.

■ The *salivary glands* produce and secrete saliva, a substance that helps with chewing and swallowing by moistening the food.

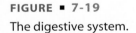

Peristalsis ■■■ involuntary wave-like muscular movements, such as those that occur in the digestive system to move chyme (partially digested food) through the intestines

- The *liver* produces and secretes *bile*, a substance that helps us to digest fat.
- The *gallbladder*, a small pouch that is attached to the liver, stores bile produced by the liver that is not secreted directly into the small intestine.
- The *pancreas produces* substances that aid in digestion and secretes them into the small intestine. The pancreas also produces insulin and glucagon, hormones that are secreted directly into the bloodstream.

Mouth

Food is taken in through the mouth. Digestion begins in the mouth. First, we physically break the food into smaller pieces by chewing it. Next, enzymes in our saliva start to work on the smaller pieces of food, breaking them down even more.

Digestion ▪▪▪ the process of breaking food down into simple elements (nutrients)

Enzymes ▪▪▪ substances that have the ability to break chemical bonds

Pharynx

From the mouth, the food moves into the pharynx (throat).

Esophagus

From the pharynx, the food passes into the esophagus, a long, narrow tube that serves mainly as a passageway for food to get from the pharynx to the stomach. The esophagus passes through the chest cavity, behind the heart. After entering the abdominal cavity, the esophagus connects with the upper part of the stomach. The mucus secreted by the esophageal mucosa, as well as the action of the muscle layer, helps to move food downward and into the stomach. The *esophageal (cardiac) sphincter*, a circle of muscular tissue, surrounds the place where the esophagus enters the stomach and keeps food from going back up the esophagus after it has entered the stomach.

Stomach

The stomach is a hollow, muscular holding pouch for food. The food we eat stays in the stomach for 3 to 4 hours, where digestion continues to take place. Special glands in the stomach lining produce stomach acid and enzymes. The stomach acid and enzymes act on the pieces of food to break them down even further. The muscular action of the stomach helps to mix the food with the acid and enzymes, creating a liquid substance called *chyme*.

Small intestine

The chyme leaves the stomach through the *pyloric sphincter*, a circle of muscular tissue that surrounds the place where the stomach empties into the small intestine and helps to prevent food from returning to the stomach once it enters the small intestine. The small intestine has three regions, called the *duodenum*, the *jejunum*, and the *ileum* (see Fig. 7-19). In the duodenum, the chyme mixes with bile (secreted by the liver) and digestive enzymes secreted by the pancreas. These substances cause further breakdown of the food.

When the chyme reaches the jejunum, absorption of nutrients begins. To reach the bloodstream, the nutrients pass through the mucosa and into the blood vessels in the submucosa. The mucosa of the small intestine has millions of tiny, finger-like structures called *villi* (Fig. 7-20). The villi increase the small intestine's ability to absorb nutrients by increasing the surface area of the mucosa.

Absorption ▪▪▪ transfer of nutrients from the digestive tract into the bloodstream

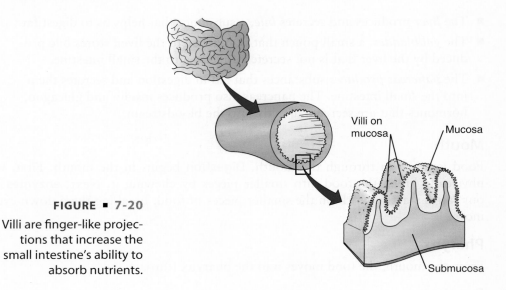

FIGURE ■ 7-20

Villi are finger-like projections that increase the small intestine's ability to absorb nutrients.

Large intestine

After leaving the ileum of the small intestine, the chyme passes into the large intestine (*colon*). The large intestine also has several distinct regions (see Fig. 7-19):

- The *cecum* is like a "waiting room" for food that is leaving the small intestine and entering the large intestine. The *appendix* is a tiny, closed pouch that dangles from the cecum. Inflammation or infection of the appendix causes *appendicitis*.
- The *ascending colon* travels upward from the cecum.
- The *transverse colon* travels across.
- The *descending colon* travels down.
- The *sigmoid colon* is an S-shaped curve at the end of the descending colon.
- The *rectum* is the last segment of the colon. The place where the rectum opens to the outside of the body is the *anus*.

Although most of the absorption of nutrients takes place in the small intestine, the large intestine also plays a role in absorption. Bacteria that live in the large intestine act on the chyme to produce vitamin K and some B vitamins, which are absorbed by the body. The action of these bacteria on the chyme can also produce gas as a by-product.

As the chyme passes slowly through the large intestine, water is absorbed into the bloodstream. By the time the chyme reaches the rectum, all nutrients and most of the water have been removed, and the chyme has taken on the consistency of normal feces. The walls of the rectum gradually expand as the feces build up. At a certain point, the brain senses that the rectum is "full" and the urge to have a bowel movement occurs.

The effects of aging on the digestive system

Difficulty chewing and swallowing

In older people, saliva production decreases, which may make chewing and swallowing more difficult. In addition, many older people have dental problems, such as missing or painful teeth. An older person may choke as a result of trying to swallow food that has not been chewed properly. Remember this when you are helping an older person to eat. Create a relaxed, social environment for eating and help the person to cut food up into small, easy-to-chew pieces.

Increased risk for constipation

In an older person, the movement of food through the digestive tract may be slower. This can put the older person at risk for constipation. The chyme spends more time in the large intestine, which allows more water to be reabsorbed into the bloodstream. As a result, by the time the chyme reaches the end of the large intestine, almost all of the water has been removed and the resulting feces are hard, dry, and difficult to pass. Certain medications (such as prescription pain relievers) and immobility can also increase a person's risk for constipation. Measures that you can take to help your patients and residents avoid constipation are described in Chapter 23.

Constipation ▪▪▪ a condition that occurs when the feces remain in the instestines for too long, resulting in hard, dry feces that are difficult to pass

Putting it all together!

- The digestive tract consists of the mouth, pharynx, esophagus, stomach, small intestine, and large intestine. The walls of the digestive tract are lined with a mucous membrane (mucosa) and contain smooth muscle, which contracts to move food through the digestive tract.

- The accessory organs of the digestive system play a role in digestion but are not actually part of the digestive tract. Accessory organs include the teeth, salivary glands, liver, gallbladder, and pancreas.

- The digestive system breaks down the food we eat into nutrients that can be used by the cells of the body. The digestive system also removes waste from the body in the form of feces. Most digestion takes place in the mouth and stomach. Most absorption takes place in the small and large intestines. Feces are what are left after all of the nutrients and most of the water have been removed from the chyme during its passage through the small and large intestines.

- As a person gets older, he or she may have more trouble chewing and swallowing food. In addition, the older person may be at higher risk for becoming constipated.

THE URINARY SYSTEM

What will you learn?

When you are finished with this section, you will be able to:

1. List and describe the main parts of the urinary system.

2. Describe the main functions of the urinary system.

3. Describe the normal changes related to aging that occur in the urinary system.

4. Define the words filtrate and urine.

Structure and function of the urinary system

The urinary system consists of the kidneys, the ureters, the bladder, and the urethra (Fig. 7-21). The main function of the urinary system is to remove waste products and excess fluid from the body. The urinary system also helps to regulate the acidity of the blood. All of these functions are essential for helping the body to maintain homeostasis.

Kidneys

We have two kidneys. Blood passes through the kidneys to be cleaned. It takes the kidneys half an hour to clean all of the blood in the body.

Inside each kidney are approximately 1 million tiny *nephrons*, which are the units that clean the blood (Fig. 7-22). Each nephron consists of a *glomerulus* and a series of *tubules*. The glomerulus is a capillary bed, located inside a structure called *Bowman's capsule*. The walls of the capillaries in the glomerulus have tiny openings in them. Because the blood is under a lot of pressure, a lot of the liquid in the blood squeezes through the walls of the capillaries, taking the wastes and nutrients that are dissolved in it with it. This liquid, called filtrate, flows into the tubules that make up the rest of the nephron. As the filtrate flows through the tubules, the capillaries reabsorb useful substances such as water, nutrients, and minerals back

Filtrate ▪▪▪ the liquid that forms the basis for urine

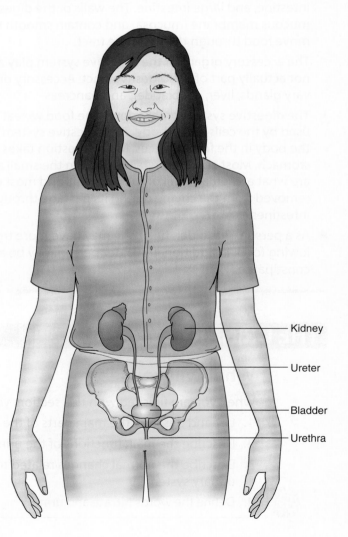

Kidney

Ureter

Bladder

Urethra

FIGURE ▪ 7-21
The urinary system.

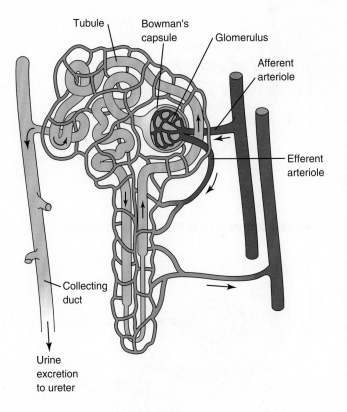

Tubule

Bowman's
capsule

Glomerulus

Afferent
arteriole

Efferent
arteriole

Collecting
duct

Urine
excretion
to ureter

FIGURE ■ 7-22

Each nephron consists of a glomerulus and a series of tubules. Blood (*red*) enters the glomerulus through the *afferent* arteriole (*afferent* means "enter"). The glomerulus filters the blood, producing filtrate, the basis of urine (*yellow*). Filtered blood (*purple*) leaves the glomerulus through the efferent arteriole (*efferent* means "exit") and is returned to the circulation.

into the bloodstream. By the time the filtrate reaches the end of the tubules, only excess fluid and waste products remain. This is urine. The kidneys produce about 1 to 1.5 liters of urine per day.

Urine ■■■ formed by the kidneys; consists of waste products that have been filtered from the bloodstream, along with excess fluid

Urine from each nephron is emptied into a collecting area called the *renal pelvis*. From the renal pelvis, the urine flows into the ureters.

Ureters

The ureters, two slender, muscular tubes, carry urine from the kidneys to the bladder. The ureters are wider at the top where they connect to the renal pelvis, but they quickly become very narrow. Where the two ureters enter the bladder, a small triangular fold of tissue called the *trigone* keeps urine from flowing back into the ureters after it has emptied into the bladder.

The ureters are lined with a mucous membrane, which helps to protect against infection. Smooth muscle in the walls of the ureters contracts rhythmically, moving urine away from the kidney and toward the bladder.

Bladder

The bladder is a hollow sac that is a holding place for urine. Like the ureters, the inside of the bladder is lined with a mucous membrane. The walls of the bladder contain three layers of smooth muscle. When the walls of the bladder contract, urination occurs. The *internal sphincter*, a ring of involuntary muscle located where the bladder and the urethra join, keeps the bladder closed while it fills. The *external urethral sphincter*, a ring of voluntary muscle, relaxes to allow urine to pass during urination.

A moderately full bladder usually contains about 1 pint (470 mL) of urine. When about 200 to 300 mL of urine collects in the bladder, the internal sphincter

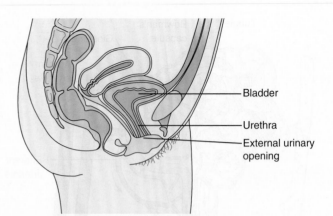

Bladder

Urethra

External urinary opening

Female urethra: 1½ to 2½ inches and straight

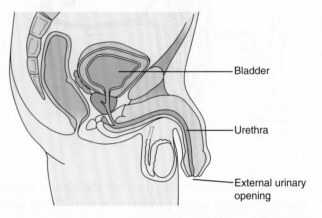

Bladder

Urethra

External urinary opening

FIGURE ▪ 7-23

Female and male urethras.   **Male urethra:** 6 to 8 inches and "S"-shaped

opens and allows urine to flood the upper part of the urethra. At this point, the urge to urinate occurs. The person voluntarily relaxes the external urethral sphincter, and the muscles of the bladder contract, allowing urine to pass out of the body through the urethra. Although it is possible to delay urination for some time, eventually the bladder will empty itself automatically.

Urethra

The urethra is the tube that carries urine from the bladder to the outside of the body. The urethra begins just below the internal sphincter and ends at the *urinary meatus*. Male and female urethras are different in size and function (Fig. 7-23). In women, the urethra is used only to pass urine. In men, the urethra serves as a passageway for both urine and semen.

The effects of aging on the urinary system

The normal processes of aging affect the urinary system in several different ways:

- **Less efficient removal of waste from the blood.** After a person reaches 40 years of age or so, the number of functioning nephrons in the kidneys starts to decrease, decreasing the kidneys' ability to filter waste products from the bloodstream.

- **Decreased muscle tone.** Loss of muscle tone as a result of aging can reduce the amount of urine the bladder can hold and may contribute to stress incontinence. This type of urinary incontinence, which is most common in older women who have had children or are obese, can often be corrected with exercises or surgery.

- **Enlargement of the prostate gland (in men).** In older men, enlargement of the prostate gland is common. As the prostate gland enlarges, it pushes against the urethra, causing it to narrow. Total emptying of the bladder of urine becomes difficult. Because the bladder does not empty completely when the man urinates, it refills with urine quickly, and the urine simply overflows. As a result, the man may "dribble" urine in between visits to the bathroom.

- **Increased risk for urinary tract infections.** Older people are also more likely to get urinary tract infections. Incomplete emptying of the bladder can contribute to the development of infections, as can a decrease in immune system functioning.

Although it is important for everyone to drink plenty of water and other fluids, it is especially important for older people. Drinking plenty of fluids helps the kidneys to work properly, and regular urination flushes harmful bacteria from the bladder, helping to prevent urinary tract infections.

Putting it all together!

- The main function of the urinary system is to remove waste products and excess fluid from the body. The urinary system also plays a role in homeostasis by regulating the acidity of the blood.

- The urinary system consists of the kidneys, the ureters, the bladder, and the urethra. The kidneys filter the blood to form urine. The ureters carry the urine from the kidneys to the bladder. The bladder is a holding place for urine. The urethra carries the urine from the bladder to the outside of the body.

- As we age, loss of muscle tone affects the bladder's ability to hold urine and empty properly, and our kidneys become less efficient at filtering the blood of waste products. In older men, enlargement of the prostate gland can lead to "dribbling" of urine. Older people are also at risk for urinary tract infections.

THE REPRODUCTIVE SYSTEM

What will you learn?

When you are finished with this section, you will be able to:

1. List and describe the main parts of the female reproductive system.
2. Discuss the main functions of the female reproductive system.
3. List and describe the main parts of the male reproductive system.
4. Discuss the main functions of the male reproductive system.

5. Describe the normal changes related to aging that occur in the reproductive system.

6. Define the words reproduction, sex cells, conception (fertilization), puberty, menopause, menstrual period, ovulation, lactation, and ejaculation.

Reproduction ■■■ the process by which a living thing makes more living things like itself

Sex cells (gametes) ■■■ special cells contributed by each parent that contain half of the normal number of chromosomes

Conception (fertilization) ■■■ occurs when the male and female sex cells join, forming a cell that contains the complete number of chromosomes

Puberty ■■■ the period during which the secondary sex characteristics appear and the reproductive organs begin to function

Menopause ■■■ the cessation of menstruation and fertility that women typically experience in their early 50s

Menstrual period ■■■ the monthly loss of blood through the vagina that occurs in the absence of pregnancy

Structure and function of the reproductive system

Without a means of reproduction, human life would cease to exist. One of the main functions of the reproductive system in both men and women is to produce and transport sex cells (gametes). Each species has a set number of genes, or chromosomes. For example, human beings have 46 chromosomes. This means that to keep the number of chromosomes the same from generation to generation, the father's sex cell (the *sperm*) contains 23 chromosomes and the mother's sex cell (the *egg* or *ovum*) contains 23 chromosomes. When the sperm joins the egg, conception (fertilization) occurs. During the 9 months leading up to the birth of a baby, the single original cell that formed at conception copies itself over and over again, forming all of the baby's tissues and organs.

The female reproductive system

The female reproductive system is designed to produce eggs, receive sperm cells, contain and nourish a developing baby, give birth, and provide nourishment after the baby's birth by producing breast milk. Each month during a woman's reproductive years (from puberty to menopause), her body prepares itself to become pregnant. If pregnancy does not occur, the woman has a menstrual period, and the cycle begins again.

INTERNAL ORGANS The internal organs of the female reproductive system are the ovaries, fallopian tubes, uterus, and vagina (Fig. 7-24).

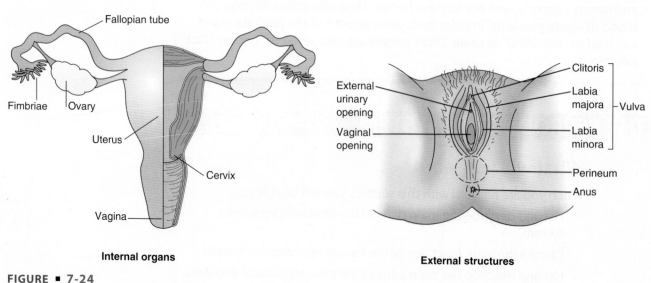

Internal organs

External structures

FIGURE ■ 7-24

The female reproductive system.

- **Ovaries.** When a girl baby is born, her ovaries contain all of the eggs she will ever have. The stored eggs are kept in a "holding pattern" until they are needed. Once a girl reaches puberty, ovulation occurs each month.
- **Fallopian tubes.** The fallopian tubes are slender tubes about 4 to 5 inches long that transport the egg from the ovary to the uterus. Fertilization, if it occurs, occurs in the fallopian tubes.
- **Uterus.** The uterus ("womb") is a hollow, muscular organ. If fertilization has occurred, the fertilized egg will attach to the lining of the uterus, called the *endometrium*, and continue to grow. (If fertilization has not occurred, the egg dissolves and is shed with the lining of the uterus during the menstrual period.) The muscular walls of the uterus expand to make room for the growing baby and then contract during labor to push the baby out. The *cervix* is the lower, narrow portion of the uterus. A very small opening allows sperm to enter and menstrual blood to leave. The cervix dilates during labor to allow a baby to be born.
- **Vagina.** The vagina is a muscular tube about 3 inches long that connects the uterus to the outside of the body. The vagina is the receiving organ for sperm. It also serves as the birth canal through which a baby passes during birth.

Ovulation ▪▪▪ the release of a ripe, mature egg from the female ovaries each month

EXTERNAL STRUCTURES The external structures of the female reproductive system, sometimes collectively referred to as the *vulva*, are the vaginal opening, the labia, and the clitoris (see Fig. 7-24).

- The **vaginal opening** is where the vagina opens to the outside of the body. The vaginal opening is located between the external urinary opening and the anus.
- The **labia**, or "lips," are folds of tissue that surround the vaginal opening.
- The **clitoris** is located at the top of the labia. This tissue, which is very sensitive to touch, helps a woman to become sexually aroused.

ACCESSORY ORGANS The breasts (mammary glands) nourish the newborn baby. Although the female breasts develop during puberty, they do not produce milk until the end of pregnancy. The breasts are made up of lobes, or sections, that contain glandular tissue and fat (Fig. 7-25). When the breast tissue is stimulated by the hormone prolactin, lactation occurs. In response to the baby's suckling, the glandular tissue contracts, sending the milk through the ducts to the nipple.

Lactation ▪▪▪ the process by which the glandular tissue of the female breast produces milk

The male reproductive system

The male reproductive system is designed to produce sperm and deposit it inside the female's body. The organs and structures of the male reproductive system include the testicles (testes), the epididymis, the vas deferens, and the penis (Fig. 7-26). Accessory organs include the seminal vesicles and prostate gland.

- **Testicles (testes).** The testicles are located in the *scrotum*, a loose, bag-like sac of skin that is suspended outside of the body between the thighs. The testicles secrete testosterone, the hormone that is responsible for the development of male secondary sex characteristics and for the proper functioning of the male reproductive system. The testicles also produce sperm cells. The testicles are located outside of a man's body because the temperature necessary for the proper development of sperm is lower than the temperature inside the body.

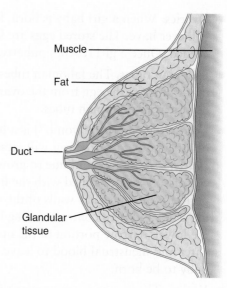

FIGURE ▪ 7-25

The breasts consist of glandular tissue and fat.

- **Epididymis.** After the sperm cells leave the testes, they move into the epididymis, a series of coiled tubes where the sperm cells mature and develop the whip-like "tail" that gives them the ability to "swim" through the female reproductive tract in search of an egg to fertilize.

- **Vas deferens.** From the epididymis, the sperm cells move into the vas deferens, a passageway that transports the sperm cells to the urethra. While in the vas deferens, the sperm cells are mixed with the secretions from the seminal vesicles and the prostate gland. These secretions, which nourish and protect the sperm cells, form *semen*, the fluid that carries the sperm cells out of the body. In the prostate gland, the vas deferens joins with the urethra, which is the final passageway through which the sperm cells leave the man's body.

- **Penis.** The male urethra is contained in the penis. Semen (and urine) leave the man's body by way of the external urinary opening, which is located at the tip of the penis. The urethra is surrounded by "spongy" tissue. Stimulation by the

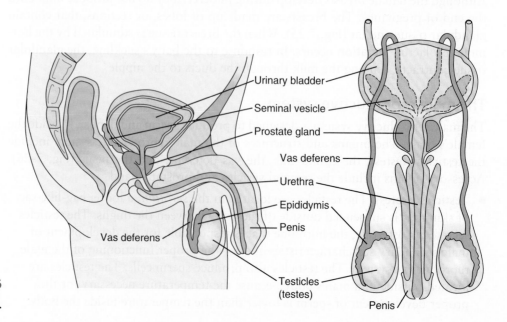

FIGURE ▪ 7-26

The male reproductive system.

nervous system causes this spongy tissue to fill with blood. This, in turn, causes the penis to become hard and erect. When erect, the penis can be inserted into a woman's vagina, allowing sperm cells to be deposited into the woman's reproductive tract via ejaculation.

Ejaculation ▪▪▪ the forceful release of semen from the body; method by which sperm cells leave the man's body through the penis

The effects of aging on the reproductive system

The female reproductive system

As a woman ages, her body produces lower amounts of sex hormones, resulting in menopause. Menopause can cause many uncomfortable symptoms, including "hot flashes," irritability, a loss of energy, and an inability to sleep. Decreased production of female sex hormones may also cause some women to develop facial hair and a coarse ("scratchy") voice. Some women experience vaginal dryness and irritation and may need to use a lubricant during sexual intercourse.

The male reproductive system

As they get older, many men find that the frequency and duration of their erections decreases. This is a result of decreased sex hormone production. A man's ability to have and maintain an erection may also be affected by the effects of aging on the cardiovascular system, which can result in decreased blood flow to the penis. Medications taken for hypertension and other common disorders can also affect a man's sexual abilities.

As a man ages, the prostate gland tends to enlarge. Because the prostate gland surrounds the urethra, this enlargement can make urination difficult. Prostate problems associated with aging are discussed earlier in this chapter.

Putting it all together!

- Reproduction is the process by which a living thing makes more living things like itself. Although in both men and women the reproductive system produces cells and hormones that are necessary to create a new life, the organs that make up the reproductive system are very different in men and women.

- The female reproductive system is designed to produce eggs, receive sperm cells, contain and nourish a developing baby, give birth, and provide nourishment after the baby's birth by producing breast milk. Each month during a woman's reproductive years, her body prepares itself to become pregnant. If pregnancy does not occur, the woman has a menstrual period, and the cycle begins again.

- The male reproductive system is designed to produce sperm and deposit it inside the female's body.

- Aging affects both the female and male reproductive systems by causing a decrease in sex hormone production. In women, this decrease results in menopause (the end of menstruation and the possibility of childbearing). In men, this decrease may make it more difficult for the man to have and maintain an erection.

What did you learn?

Multiple Choice

Select the single best answer for each of the following questions.

1. What is the purpose of epithelial tissue?
   a. To provide a frame for, and give shape to, the body.
   b. To connect other types of tissue together
   c. To cover the body and line its cavities
   d. To conduct nerve impulses

2. The substance found in the epidermis that gives our skin, hair, and eyes color is called:
   a. Keratin
   b. Melanin
   c. Sebum
   d. Collagen

3. Which of the following is a normal age-related change affecting the integumentary system?
   a. The nails become thick and tough
   b. The body produces less sweat
   c. The skin becomes dry and fragile
   d. All of the above

4. Which of the following is a function of the skeletal system?
   a. It acts as a storage site for vitamin C
   b. It produces heat
   c. It produces blood cells
   d. All of the above

5. When a muscle atrophies, it becomes:
   a. Larger and stronger
   b. Thinner and weaker
   c. Stiff
   d. More flexible

6. Where does gas exchange take place in the respiratory system?
   a. In the alveoli
   b. In the bronchioles
   c. In the pharynx
   d. In the nasal cavity

7. What part of the respiratory tract is also known as the "windpipe"?
   a. Pharynx
   b. Epiglottis
   c. Larynx
   d. Trachea

8. The upper chambers of the heart are called the:
   a. Ventricles
   b. Atria
   c. Mitral valves
   d. Arterioles

9. Blood cells that contain hemoglobin and carry oxygen are called:
   a. Leukocytes
   b. Phagocytes
   c. Thrombocytes
   d. Erythrocytes

10. Varicose veins are commonly caused by:
    a. Loss of elasticity in the veins
    b. Forceful heart contractions
    c. Loss of elasticity in the arteries
    d. A decreased number of red blood cells

11. How does aging affect the nervous system?
    a. Older people usually become "senile" and forgetful
    b. Older people lose the ability to form or understand words
    c. Older people may take slightly longer to react to things
    d. Aging does not affect the nervous system because old neurons are constantly replaced

12. What is the fatty white substance covering a nerve fiber that helps speed the conduction of nerve impulses?
    a. Meninges
    b. Synapse
    c. Myelin
    d. Dendrite

13. What is the largest part of the brain?
    a. Cerebrum
    b. Cerebellum
    c. Brain stem
    d. Diencephalon

14. As a normal part of aging, many older people gradually lose the ability to hear high-pitched sounds. What is this called?
    a. Presbyopia
    b. Presbycusis
    c. Vestibular apparatus
    d. Cerumen

15. Hormones are chemical messengers that allow the body to:
    a. Metabolize energy
    b. Grow
    c. Reproduce
    d. All of the above

16. What hormone is secreted by the pancreas to help the body manage blood sugar levels?
    a. Insulin
    b. Thyroxine
    c. Glucocorticoids
    d. Antidiuretic hormone (ADH)

17. What is another term for the large intestine?
    a. Stomach
    b. Duodenum
    c. Cecum
    d. Colon

18. Bile helps to break down fats. Where is bile produced?
    a. Pancreas
    b. Liver
    c. Stomach
    d. Salivary glands

19. Normal changes in the digestive system related to aging include:
    a. More difficulty chewing and swallowing
    b. Sharper sense of taste and increased appetite
    c. Decreased risk for constipation
    d. All of the above

20. The tube that connects the kidneys to the bladder is called the:
    a. Ureter
    b. Urethra
    c. Trigone
    d. Sphincter

21. How much urine does an average adult pass each day?
    a. 200 mL of urine
    b. 500 mL of urine
    c. 1 to 1.5 liters of urine
    d. 160 to 180 liters of urine

22. How does aging affect the urinary system?
    a. The kidneys' ability to filter waste from the blood decreases
    b. The bladder is able to hold more urine
    c. The person's risk for constipation is increased
    d. The person's urine becomes darker

23. The complete ending of a woman's menstrual cycle that commonly occurs as part of the aging process is called:
    a. Puberty
    b. Pregnancy
    c. Menstrual period
    d. Menopause

24. What occurs when a male sex cell joins the female sex cell, forming a cell that contains the complete number of chromosomes?
    a. Ovulation
    b. Menstruation
    c. Menopause
    d. Conception

25. Where does conception usually occur?
    a. In the uterus
    b. In the vagina
    c. In the fallopian tube
    d. In the vas deferens

Matching

Match each organ system with its description.

_____ 1. Musculoskeletal system

_____ 2. Reproductive system

_____ 3. Endocrine system

_____ 4. Integumentary system

_____ 5. Digestive system

_____ 6. Respiratory system

_____ 7. Nervous system

_____ 8. Urinary system

_____ 9. Sensory system

_____ 10. Cardiovascular system

a. Provides a covering to protect the body

b. Allows the body to move

c. Provides oxygen and removes carbon dioxide

d. Transports oxygen and nutrients to the cells of the body

e. Receives, processes, and stores information

f. Protects us from harm and lets us experience the world we live in through the senses of touch, taste, sight, smell, and hearing

g. Controls body functions by secretion of hormones

h. Processes food and rids the body of waste

i. Filters the blood to remove excess fluid and waste

j. Provides the ability to produce children

 Stop and Think!

One of your residents, Mr. Conrad, has been suffering from a lung disorder for many years. He has difficulty breathing and seems to be prone to catch pneumonia. After learning about the function of the respiratory system, explain what effect a breathing disorder has on Mr. Conrad's body. What other body systems could this affect?

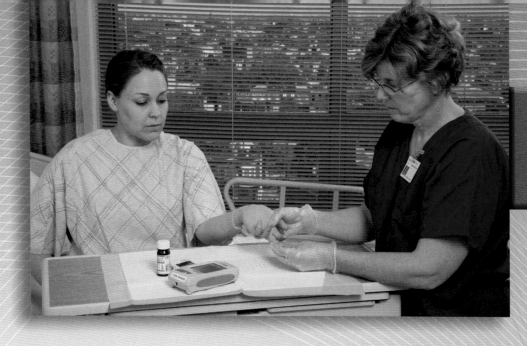

CHAPTER 8

The nursing assistant checks the blood glucose level of a patient with diabetes, a disorder that occurs when the body is not able to produce or respond to the hormone insulin.

Common Disorders

Illnesses and injuries that result in disability are the main reasons a person will need the type of care that nursing assistants provide. You have learned about how the body functions when it is healthy. Now you will learn more about what happens to the body's organ systems as a result of illness or injury.

INTRODUCTION TO DISORDERS

What will you learn?

When you are finished with this section, you will be able to:

1. Discuss the difference between acute and chronic disorders.
2. Describe the general categories used to describe the causes of disorders.
3. List factors that may put a person for risk for developing a certain disorder.

4. Define the words disease, acute, and chronic.

Disease ▪▪▪ a condition that occurs when the structure or function of an organ or organ system is abnormal

Acute ▪▪▪ a word used to describe a disorder with a rapid onset and a relatively short recovery time; usually unexpected

Chronic ▪▪▪ a word used to describe a disorder that is ongoing and often needs to be controlled through continuous medication or treatment

A disorder is something that affects the body's ability to maintain homeostasis. A disorder may also be called a "disease" or an "illness." A disorder can be acute or chronic. Disorders can be grouped into several broad categories based on their causes (Table 8-1).

Many factors can put a person at risk for developing a disorder or negatively affect his ability to recover from a disorder (Box 8-1). Awareness of the factors that can put your patients or residents at risk for a disorder will help you to better meet their individual needs.

TABLE 8-1	Types of Disorders	
TYPE OF DISORDER	**CAUSE**	**EXAMPLES**
Infectious	Germs invade the body	Pneumonia, urinary tract infections, AIDS
Degenerative	The tissues of the body wear out or break down	Arthritis, osteoporosis, Alzheimer's disease
Nutritional	The person's diet is out of balance	Obesity, malnutrition
Metabolic (endocrine)	The body is unable to metabolize or absorb certain nutrients; often the result of producing too much of one type of hormone or not enough	Diabetes
Immunologic	The immune system does not work properly; the immune system may not be able to fight off infection, or the immune system starts to attack the body's own tissues	AIDS, rheumatoid arthritis, multiple sclerosis
Neoplastic	A tumor invades otherwise healthy tissues and prevents the tissues from functioning properly	Cancer
Psychiatric (mental)	The person is unable to maintain emotional balance	Depression, schizophrenia
Traumatic	The body's ability to function is changed by an outside force	Accidents, gunshot wounds, stabbing

Box 8-1   Risk Factors for Disorders

- **Age.** Some disorders are more likely to occur in certain age groups. Age can also influence how a person reacts to disease. For example, an older person is much more likely to experience complications from the flu than a younger person is.

- **Gender.** Some disorders are more common in men than in women, and vice versa. For example, women are more likely to develop breast cancer than men are.

- **Heredity.** The genes that we get from our parents may put us at risk for developing certain diseases. For example, scientists now know that some types of cancer, diabetes, and heart disease are inherited.

- **Lifestyle.** A person's living conditions and health habits play a major role in the person's overall health status. For example, a person who smokes is more likely to develop cancer, lung disease, or heart disease than a person who does not.

- **Occupation.** Many jobs put a person at risk for certain diseases. For example, health care workers who do not take care to protect themselves are at risk for certain infections, such as human immunodeficiency virus (HIV) or hepatitis.

- **Chronic disease.** A person who has a chronic disease, such as diabetes or high blood pressure, is at increased risk for developing another disease. In addition, a person who has a chronic disease may be more likely to experience more severe problems from something that would not really affect a healthy person.

- **Emotional stress.** A person's emotional health can directly affect his or her physical health. Emotional stress can create physical problems such as headaches and digestive disorders, and it puts the body at higher risk for infection.

Putting it all together!

- When the body's ability to maintain homeostasis is altered, a disorder can result. A disorder can be acute (temporary) or chronic (long term).
- A disorder can be described as infectious, degenerative, nutritional, metabolic, immunologic, neoplastic, psychiatric, or traumatic in origin.
- Being aware of the factors that put a person at risk for disease will help you to provide better care for your patients or residents because you will have a better understanding of each individual's needs.

INTEGUMENTARY DISORDERS

What will you learn?

When you are finished with this section, you will be able to:

1. Describe how an integumentary system disorder can place a person at risk for infection.
2. Describe what a burn is, and list the different types of burns.

TELL THE NURSE !

SIGNS AND SYMPTOMS OF INTEGUMENTARY DISORDERS

- There is a new rash or changes in an existing rash
- There is a new bruise
- The skin looks abnormally pale or flushed or has a bluish or yellowish hue
- A mole has changed in appearance
- A wound that will not heal

3. Describe what a lesion is, and list the different types of lesions.

4. Discuss actions a nursing assistant can take to help promote comfort and skin healing in a person with a skin lesion.

5. Define the words lesion and rash.

Many people in your care will have a disorder of the integumentary system. Sometimes, this disorder is the reason the person is in the health care facility. For example, this might be the case for a person who has suffered severe burns or trauma. Other times, the disorder develops after the person is already in the health care facility. For example, a person might develop a pressure ulcer or have surgery that results in a surgical wound that must heal. Any break in the skin can allow germs to invade the body and cause an infection. If one of your patients or residents develops any type of skin disorder, you will need to report this to the nurse quickly so that measures can be taken to help the skin to heal and to prevent infection.

Pressure ulcers

Pressure ulcers may form if a person is not able to move freely on his or her own. Pressure ulcers are discussed in detail in Chapter 19.

Burns

Burns are injuries to the skin and underlying tissues caused by contact with extreme heat, chemicals, or electricity. Burns are classified according to the depth of the damage:

- **Superficial (First-degree) burns** cause injury to the outermost layer of the skin, the epidermis.

- **Partial-thickness (Second-degree) burns** extend into the dermis. The loss of the epidermis increases the risk of infection.

- **Full-thickness (Third-degree) burns** involve the epidermis and dermis, the subcutaneous layer, and often the underlying muscles and bones as well. Serious complications of third-degree burns include infection, scarring, and contractures (loss of motion in a joint resulting from shortening of the tendons).

People with second- and third-degree burns need very special care. Because of the risk of infection, caregivers must often wear sterile gloves and gowns when providing care, and bed linens may need to be sterilized before the bed is made.

Lesions

Lesion ▪▪▪ a general term used to describe any break in the skin

Rash ▪▪▪ a group of skin lesions

A lesion is a break in the skin (Table 8-2). Lesions often occur in groups, forming a rash. Rashes can be *localized* (limited to one area) or *systemic* (occurring all over the body). Rashes are often caused by an infection, such as chickenpox or the measles. In this case, the skin itself is not infected, but it is showing signs of an infection inside of the body. Shingles (herpes zoster), is a skin rash most commonly seen in people older than 65. It is caused by the same virus that causes chickenpox. A person with shingles should only be cared for by someone who has already been exposed to the chickenpox virus. It is possible to get chickenpox from a person with shingles if you have not been exposed to the virus before.

TABLE 8-2	**Types of Skin Lesions**
LESION	**DESCRIPTION**
 **Macule** ©Dr. P. Marazzi/Science Photo Library/ Custom Medical Stock Photo	Small, flat, red lesions
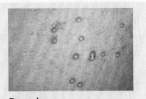 **Papule** ©Custom Medical Stock Photo	Small, raised, firm bumps
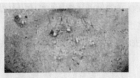 **Vesicle**	Small, fluid-filled, blister-like lesions
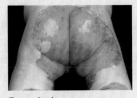 **Pustule**	Small, pus-filled, blister-like lesions
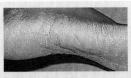 **Excoriation** ©Custom Medical Stock Photo	Abrasion (wearing away of the surface of the skin)
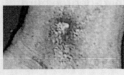 **Fissure**	A crack in the skin
Ulcer	A crater-like open sore

Guidelines Box 8-1 Guidelines for Caring for a Person With a Skin Lesion

What you do	Why you do it
Check with the nurse or consult the nursing care plan to ensure that you are aware of any changes to the normal bathing and skin care routine that may be necessary.	*A special soap or lotion may have been ordered by the doctor as part of the person's treatment for the lesion. Or a product that is used as part of the normal bathing and skin care routine may be contributing to the skin problem and should no longer be used on the person.*
Help the person to choose clothing that does not rub or irritate the skin lesion.	*Protecting the lesion from additional irritation, such as that caused by clothing rubbing against it, is important to help it heal.*
Discourage the person from scratching itchy or irritated skin.	*Although scratching may bring temporary relief, it causes additional skin injury and puts the person at risk for infection.*
Observe the lesions for changes in color or for bleeding or drainage. Also note whether the lesions seem to be getting larger or spreading to other parts of the body. Report any changes to the nurse immediately.	*Your prompt reporting of any changes that you notice will help to ensure that the person receives the proper treatment.*
Make sure to follow your facility's infection control procedures when giving care to people who have skin lesions caused by an infection such as shingles or a localized infection.	*Following the proper infection control procedures will help to prevent the spread of the infection to other patients and residents and also to the people providing care to the person.*

Rashes may also be caused by contact with an irritant, such as poison ivy, bath soap, or laundry detergent. Itching, burning, or redness of the skin accompanies many skin lesions. When you are caring for a person with skin lesions, there are several things that you can do to increase the person's comfort and promote healing of the skin (Guidelines Box 8-1).

Putting it all together!

- A break in the skin, such as that caused by wounds, burns, or lesions, puts the person at risk for infection.
- Burns are injuries caused by heat, chemicals, or electricity. Burns can be classified as first-degree (superficial), second-degree (partial-thickness) or third-degree (full-thickness) burns. People with second- and third-degree burn wounds require special care because of the very high risk of infection.
- Skin lesions can be caused by infections inside the body, infections of the skin itself, or irritation of the skin.
- As a nursing assistant, you will play a very important role in preventing the development of skin disorders, observing signs and symptoms of skin disorders, and helping people with skin disorders to heal.

MUSCULOSKELETAL DISORDERS

What will you learn?

When you are finished with this section, you will be able to:

1. Describe what osteoporosis is, and how to care for a person who has osteoporosis.

2. Describe three common types of arthritis.

3. Describe how to care for a person who has had hip-joint replacement surgery.

4. Describe how muscular dystrophy can cause disability.

5. Describe two ways that fractures are repaired, and discuss how to care for a person who has a cast.

6. Describe situations that can lead to amputation.

 7. Define the terms osteoporosis, arthritis, fracture, traction, amputation, and phantom pain.

Osteoporosis

Although everyone experiences some loss of bone tissue as a normal part of aging, people with osteoporosis lose excessive amounts of bone tissue, causing the bones to become crumbly and very fragile. The bones most commonly affected by osteoporosis are the bones of the spine (Fig. 8-1), the pelvis, and the long bones in the arms and legs.

Osteoporosis is most common in older women. Other risk factors for the development of osteoporosis include:

- White race
- "Small bones"
- Smoking
- Inactivity or immobility
- Diseases of the thyroid and adrenal glands
- A diet lacking in calcium, vitamin D (necessary for the absorption of calcium), and protein
- Certain drugs, such as steroids

Osteoporosis causes bones to break more easily, and physical activity becomes very difficult. Guidelines for caring for a person with osteoporosis are given in Guidelines Box 8-2.

Osteoporosis ▪▪▪ a disorder characterized by the excessive loss of bone tissue

Arthritis

There are many different types of arthritis. Three of the most common types are osteoarthritis, rheumatoid arthritis, and gout.

Arthritis ▪▪▪ inflammation of the joints, usually associated with pain and stiffness

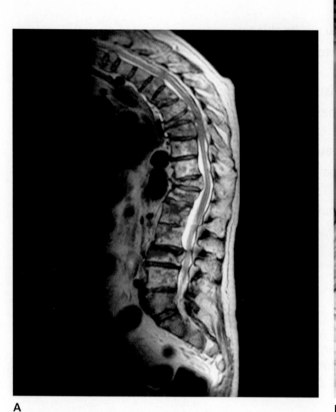

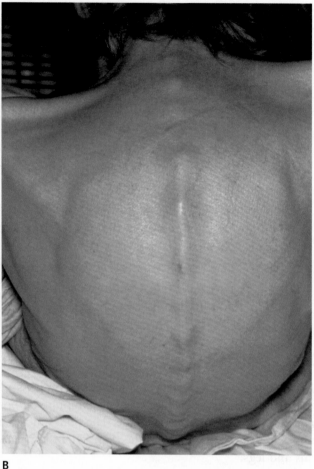

A   B

FIGURE ▪ 8-1

Osteoporosis. **(A)** A magnetic resonance imaging (MRI) scan of the spine of a 60-year-old patient with osteoporosis. This is a side view (the patient is standing, facing the left). The vertebrae (*brown*) enclose the spinal cord (*pink*). Some of the vertebrae (*orange*) have collapsed as a result of osteoporosis, causing the spine to curve. **(B)** This woman has a "dowager's hump" as a result of osteoporosis of the spine. The deformity occurs when the fragile bones of the spine crumble.

A, ©Zephyr/Photo Researchers, Inc.; B, ©John Radcliffe Hospital/Photo Researchers, Inc.

Osteoarthritis

Osteoarthritis is the leading cause of physical disability among elderly people. In osteoarthritis, the cartilage that covers the ends of the bones wears away, making movement of the joint difficult and painful. Osteoarthritis appears to be the result of normal wear and tear on the joint, which is why it is seen most often in elderly people. However, obesity, previous joint injury, or a family history of the disease may increase a person's risk of developing osteoarthritis earlier in life and more severely. Osteoarthritis usually affects weight-bearing joints, such as the knees, hips, and joints of the spine.

A person with osteoarthritis may take medications to decrease both the pain and swelling. Heat and cold applications, discussed in Chapter 24, can also increase a person's level of comfort. Mild exercise that places the affected joints through their range of motion helps to decrease stiffness and maintain joint function.

Guidelines Box 8-2   Guidelines for Caring for a Person With Osteoporosis

What you do	Why you do it
Remember to be gentle when helping the person to move.	*Sometimes bones are so brittle that a person can break them just by bumping into a piece of furniture. Bones that break are difficult to repair and heal slowly.*
Encourage exercise by having the person take frequent walks with you.	*Exercise helps to strengthen the bones and prevent complications of immobility.*
Carefully observe and document the types of foods and liquids the person eats and drinks, and encourage snacks that are high in calcium, such as milk, yogurt, ice cream, and cheese.	*Additional calcium can help slow bone loss.*
Be especially observant of loss of function, swelling, or complaints of pain.	*These signs and symptoms may indicate that a fragile bone has broken.*

People who have very severe osteoarthritis may need joint replacement surgery, which involves removing the ends of the bones in the affected joint and replacing them with parts made from metal and plastic (Fig. 8-2). Hip and knee replacements are most common. Guidelines for caring for a person who has had hip replacement surgery are given in Guidelines Box 8-3.

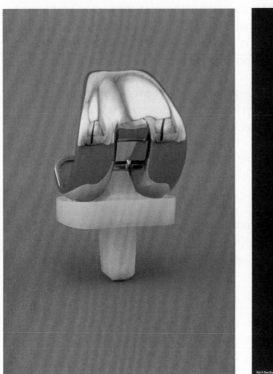

A

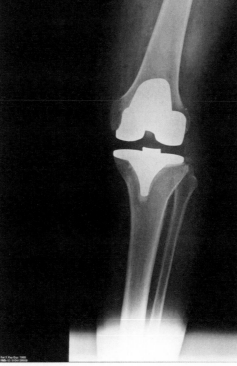

B

FIGURE ■ 8-2

In joint replacement surgery, a damaged joint is replaced with an artificial (prosthetic) joint. **(A)** An artificial knee joint. **(B)** X-ray of an artificial knee joint in place.

A, ©SIU Bio Med/Custom Medical Stock Photo.

Guidelines Box 8-3 Guidelines for Caring for a Person Who Has Had Hip Replacement Surgery

What you do	Why you do it
Assist the person with getting in and out of bed as necessary. Do not allow the person to bear weight on the affected joint without the doctor's approval.	People who have had a joint replaced are not allowed to bear weight on the affected joint for a period of time after the surgery. The ligaments are weak, and placing weight on the joint can cause the joint to "give out."
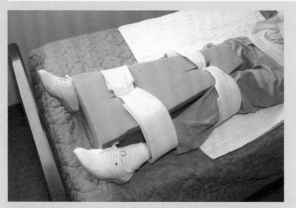 Use an abduction pillow to keep the person's legs abducted (spread apart) when the person is lying on his or her back or side.	After the surgery, the muscles and ligaments that normally hold the hip joint in place are weak, making it very easy for the head of the femur (the thigh bone) to dislocate or pop out of joint. Keeping the legs abducted when the person is lying on his or her back or side helps to prevent this.
Provide the person with a straight-backed chair to sit in.	To prevent dislocation of the joint, the person's hips must be flexed no more than 90 degrees and the person's feet must rest flat on the floor. A straight-backed chair helps to ensure the proper sitting position.
When assisting the person with elimination, use a special device to raise the height of the toilet seat, if necessary.	Raising the height of the toilet seat helps to prevent flexion of the hip joint in excess of 90 degrees when the person is using the toilet.
Ask to be present while the physical therapist is working with the person.	This will enable you to learn the proper way to assist your patient or resident with getting in and out of bed and walking.
Provide emotional support and encouragement.	Recovering from surgery can be a long, difficult, and painful process. Your reassurance and encouragement are necessary to help keep the patient or resident focused on recovery.

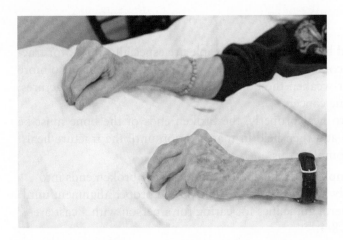

FIGURE ▪ 8-3

This woman has rheumatoid arthritis in the joints of her hands.

Rheumatoid arthritis

Rheumatoid arthritis can cause severe joint deformities (Fig. 8-3). Researchers believe that rheumatoid arthritis is an autoimmune disorder. In autoimmune disorders, the body's immune system begins to attack the body's own tissues. So, for example, in rheumatoid arthritis, the immune system attacks and destroys the cartilage that covers the ends of the bones. Scar tissue develops within the joints, causing them to become stiff and useless. For many months, a person's rheumatoid arthritis may seem to be under control, but then the person will experience an acute flare-up of the disease. During the acute phases of the disease, the person may experience pain, swelling, redness, and heat in the joints, as well as fever and general weakness. Bed rest may be necessary, and splints can help decrease joint deformity. The gentle use of range-of-motion exercises (discussed in Chapter 15) helps to maintain joint mobility.

Gout

Gout is a type of arthritis caused by a disturbance in the body's metabolism. Uric acid, a waste product that is usually eliminated by the kidneys, builds up in the body. The uric acid forms crystals in the joints and causes inflammation and pain. While gout can affect any joint, the big toe is most commonly affected. Men past middle age are more commonly affected than women.

Muscular dystrophy

Muscular dystrophy is a general term for a group of disorders that cause the skeletal muscles to become progressively weaker over time. These disorders are inherited. Some people with muscular dystrophy experience only moderate disability, while others may die from the disease. *Duchenne's muscular dystrophy* is the most common form of muscular dystrophy. It develops during childhood and usually causes death by the age of 20 years.

Myotonic muscular dystrophy is the most common type that affects adults. Myotonic muscular dystrophy causes a person to have difficulty relaxing the muscles after contracting them, and the muscles may spasm. Muscular dystrophy is a common reason why a younger person may become a resident of a long-term care facility.

Fractures

Fracture ▪▪▪ a broken bone

A fracture is usually caused by trauma. Older people are especially at risk for fractures because the bones become more fragile with age. Older people are also more likely to have diseases that weaken the bones and put them at risk for fractures, such as osteoporosis or bone cancer.

For a fractured bone to heal properly, the broken ends of the bone must be brought together (aligned) and then held in that position until the fracture heals. There are two ways to accomplish this:

- If the fracture is not complicated, the doctor can move the broken ends into alignment and then apply a cast to keep the bone in the proper alignment until it heals (Fig. 8-4A). General guidelines for caring for a person with a cast are given in Guidelines Box 8-4.

- If the fracture is complicated, surgery may be necessary, and metal plates, screws, rods, pins, or wires may be used to hold the broken ends of the bone in alignment (Fig. 8-4B).

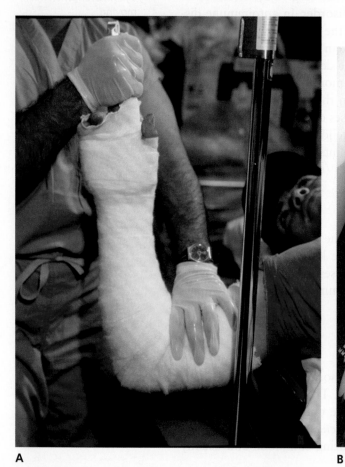
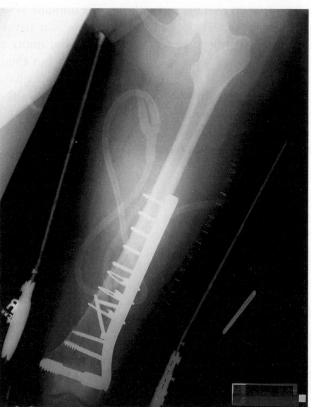

A   B

FIGURE ▪ 8-4

With any fracture, the broken ends of the bone need to be brought back together and then held in place so that healing can occur. The bone ends can be held together externally, using a cast **(A)**, or internally, using devices such as plates, screws, pins, or wires **(B)**.

A, ©L. Steinmark/Custom Medical Stock Photo.

Guidelines Box 8-4   Guidelines for Caring for a Person With a Cast

What you do	Why you do it
Do not cover the cast or place it on a plastic-covered pillow until it has dried completely.	*The casting material produces heat as it dries. Covering the cast can cause the person's skin underneath the cast to burn.*
Do not touch the cast with your fingertips until it is totally dry. If you must handle the cast, use the palms of your hands.	*Touching the cast can cause it to dent, creating pressure spots against the person's skin.*
Keep the casted body part elevated on a pillow for several days.	*Elevating the casted body part helps prevent and reduce swelling around the fracture site.*
Because the skin underneath the cast can start to itch, the person may try to slide an object between the cast and the skin in order to scratch the itchy area. Advise the person that placing objects inside of the cast should be avoided.	*Sliding an object between the cast and the skin may injure the skin, which puts the person at risk for infection.*
Make sure the person's toes (or fingers, if the cast is on the arm) are pink, warm, and moving. Report any complaints of increased pain, numbness, or tingling. Report any observations of cyanosis, increased swelling, cold toes or fingers, increased drainage on the cast, or a foul odor immediately.	*Cyanosis; increased swelling; increased pain, numbness, or tingling; or cold fingers or toes may indicate that swelling inside the cast is interfering with blood flow. If the tissues do not receive enough oxygen and nutrients, tissue death and skin breakdown may occur. Increased drainage or a foul odor may indicate infection.*
Keep the cast clean and dry.	*Plaster cast material becomes soft again when it becomes wet.*
Do not allow the person to place pressure or weight on the cast unless he or she has been specifically instructed to do so.	*Placing too much pressure or weight on the cast can cause the cast to break.*
Regularly inspect the condition of the cast and the skin around the edges of the cast.	*A crack in the cast can cause the cast to become loose or break, which could delay healing of the bone. Rough edges on the cast can irritate or break the skin, putting the person at risk for infection and other problems.*

Some fractured bones cannot be repaired surgically for a period of time, especially if the person's overall medical condition is unstable. In these cases, **traction** is used to keep the broken ends of the bone in alignment until the fracture can be permanently repaired by surgery or casting. When you are caring for a person who is in traction, be careful not to disturb the weights attached to the traction unit. When you lower the person's bed height, check to make sure the weights are not resting on the floor. They must hang freely to apply the correct amount of tension.

Traction ▪▪▪ a treatment for fracture in which the ends of the broken bone are placed in the proper alignment, and then weight is applied to exert a constant pull and keep the bone in alignment

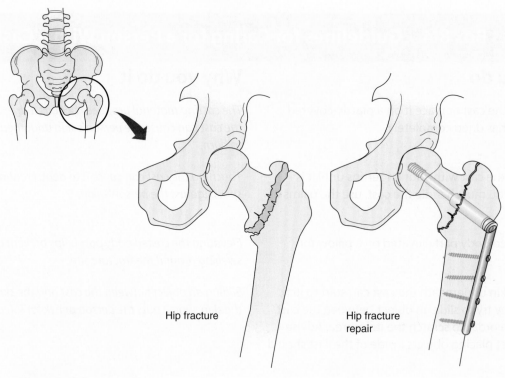

FIGURE ■ 8-5

A hip fracture is a fracture that occurs at the top of the femur (the thigh bone). The fracture is often repaired using plates, pins, and screws.

Hip fractures

Nursing assistants who work in a long-term care facility are very likely to care for people recovering from hip fractures. A *hip fracture* is a fracture that occurs at the top of the femur (thigh bone) (Fig. 8-5). Hip fractures are common in elderly people because they have an increased risk of falling and having fragile bones.

Most hip fractures are surgically reduced and stabilized with the use of plates, screws, or pins. Some people may also require joint replacement with an artificial (prosthetic) joint. During the recovery period, the person will need extensive rehabilitation to help regain strength and mobility.

Amputations

Amputation ▪▪▪ the surgical removal of all or part of an extremity

Amputation may be necessary as a result of trauma or disease. Diabetes-related foot problems are very common and account for many amputations in the United States. The loss of a body part, especially an arm or leg, is very emotionally traumatic for a person. The person's mobility, appearance, and sometimes even ability to earn a living or enjoy a hobby he or she used to love can be affected by an amputation. For some people who have had a body part either partially or completely amputated, a prosthetic (false) part may allow the person to regain mobility, function, and a more normal appearance (Fig. 8-6).

Phantom pain ▪▪▪ the feeling that a body part is still present, after it has been surgically removed (amputated)

Many people experience phantom pain after an amputation. Aching, itching, and other sensations are all types of phantom pain. The sensations are caused by the healing of the nerves that were cut when the body part was removed. Phantom pain usually goes away a short while after surgery, but some people report having these episodes for years afterward.

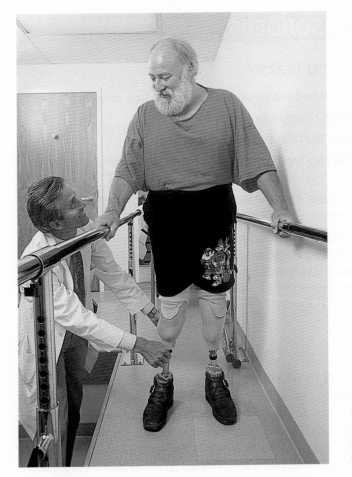

FIGURE ▪ 8-6
A prosthetic body part can help a person who has had an amputation regain function and mobility.

Putting it all together!

- Disorders of the musculoskeletal system can make mobility difficult.
- Osteoporosis is the excessive loss of bone tissue, resulting in bones that break very easily.
- Arthritis is inflammation of the joints. Osteoarthritis typically affects older adults and causes the cartilage covering the ends of the bones to become worn. People with osteoarthritis may eventually require joint replacement surgery. Rheumatoid arthritis typically affects younger people and can cause severe joint deformities.
- Gout is the build-up of uric acid that causes crystals to form in the joints. This causes inflammation and pain.
- Muscular dystrophy causes the skeletal muscles to become progressively weaker over time. Muscular dystrophy is a common reason why a younger person may become a resident of a long-term care facility.
- Older people are especially at risk for fractures, and fractures may take longer to heal in an older person. Fractures may be treated by casting or by surgical placement of plates, screws, pins, or wires.
- Amputation may become necessary because of trauma or because of complications related to a medical condition, such as diabetes.

RESPIRATORY DISORDERS

What will you learn?

When you are finished with this section, you will be able to:

1. Describe three respiratory tract infections.
2. Describe how to collect a sputum specimen.
3. Describe the two types of chronic obstructive pulmonary disease (COPD).
4. List some general care measures that a nursing assistant may use to assist a person with a respiratory disorder.
5. Define the words pneumonia, sputum, bronchitis, influenza, asthma, chronic obstructive pulmonary disease (COPD), emphysema, and chronic bronchitis.

Infections

Pneumonia

Pneumonia **■■■** inflammation of the lung tissue, caused by infection with a virus or bacterium, and resulting in impaired gas exchange

Pneumonia causes the alveoli to fill with fluid and pus, which prevents air from entering the alveoli. As a result, gas exchange (the transfer of oxygen into the blood and carbon dioxide out of it) cannot occur. Signs and symptoms of pneumonia include fever, pain when breathing, cyanosis (bluish skin as a result of decreased oxygen levels in the blood), and a productive cough. A productive cough is one in which a person coughs up sputum. You may be asked to assist in the diagnosis of pneumonia by collecting a sputum specimen for analysis (Guidelines Box 8-5).

Sputum **■■■** mucus and other respiratory secretions that are coughed up from the lungs, bronchi, and trachea; also known as *phlegm*

There are many things you can do to help a person with respiratory problems, such as pneumonia, feel more comfortable:

- Raising the head of the bed so that the person can sit up in bed is often helpful. Some people are more comfortable when they assume a forward-leaning position using pillows on the over-bed table (Fig. 8-7).

- If the doctor has not placed any restrictions on the person's fluid intake, encourage the person to drink plenty of fluids. Fluids help to thin respiratory secretions so that they are easier to cough up.

- Providing frequent oral care will also help keep the person comfortable and will reduce the number of germs that are present in the mouth.

Bronchitis

Bronchitis **■■■** inflammation of the bronchi

Bronchitis may cause a dry, nonproductive cough that sounds like a "bark." Bronchitis can turn into pneumonia if the bronchial infection is not treated promptly.

Influenza

Influenza **■■■** an acute respiratory infection caused by the influenza virus; characterized by a sore throat, dry cough, stuffy nose, headache, body aches, weakness, and fever; commonly known as "the flu"

Influenza is very contagious. Most people who get influenza will recover in about a week. However, elderly people, very young children, and people with chronic illnesses who get influenza are at risk for developing serious complications, such as an extremely severe form of pneumonia. Residents of long-term care facilities are especially at risk for experiencing complications from influenza. An annual

Guidelines Box 8-5   Guidelines for Collecting a Sputum Specimen

What you do	Why you do it
Explain to the person that the sputum for the specimen should be coughed up from deep down in the respiratory tract.	*The sputum for analysis must come from the lungs because that is where most of the infection-causing germs are located. Explaining this to the person helps to ensure that she produces a specimen that will result in an accurate diagnosis. If you do not explain this to the person she may just cough up saliva, which will not result in an accurate diagnosis.*
Provide privacy.	*Having to spit mucus into a cup can be embarrassing and unpleasant for some people.*
Have the person rinse her mouth with water before coughing up the specimen.	*Rinsing with plain water helps to remove germs that are normally present in the mouth, resulting in a "cleaner" specimen.*
Do not have the person rinse with mouthwash before coughing up the specimen.	*The antiseptic effects of the mouthwash might kill the germs in the sputum specimen that are responsible for the infection, which will result in inaccurate test results.*
Have the person spit the specimen directly into a sterile specimen container and close the lid.	*Having the person spit directly into the sterile specimen container reduces the risk of contaminating the specimen and results in more accurate test results.*
Make sure that the specimen container is labeled properly and that the information is correct.	*Labeling errors can result in misdiagnosis or the need to repeat the test.*
Take the specimen container to the laboratory immediately after collecting the specimen or ask the nurse how to store it.	*Allowing a specimen to sit around or storing it the incorrect way can result in the need to repeat the test.*

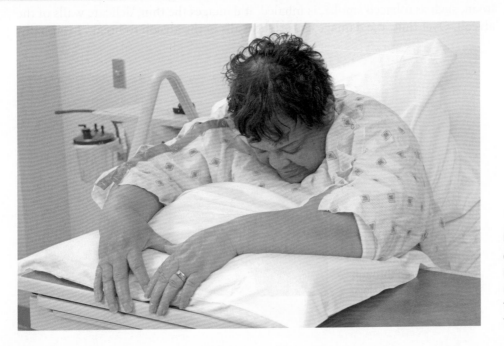

FIGURE ■ 8-7

Certain positions make breathing easier for people with respiratory disorders. Many people find that leaning forward helps to make breathing easier.

Asthma ■■■ a condition that affects the bronchi and bronchioles of the lungs; triggers (such as cold weather, allergies, respiratory infections, stress, smoke, and exercise) cause the bronchi and bronchioles to become narrower, making breathing difficult

Chronic obstructive pulmonary disease (COPD) ■■■ a general term used to describe two related lung disorders, emphysema and chronic bronchitis; the leading cause of COPD is smoking

Emphysema ■■■ a disorder caused by long-term exposure of the alveoli to toxins, such as tobacco smoke; one of two forms of chronic obstructive pulmonary disease (COPD)

FIGURE ■ 8-8

Flu shots are usually given to residents in the fall, before the start of flu season (November through April). Flu shots help to prevent infection with the influenza virus, which is very contagious and can cause serious complications in elderly people, very young children, and people with chronic illnesses.

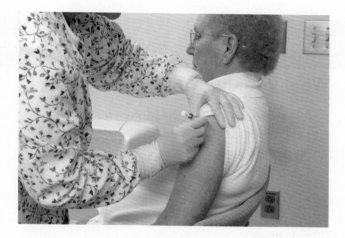

"flu shot" for both staff members and residents can help to prevent outbreaks of influenza in long-term care facilities (Fig. 8-8).

Asthma

Asthma is a chronic disorder. When a person with asthma has an asthma attack, it can be very frightening for the person because breathing becomes almost impossible. A person with asthma may need to take medications on a regular basis to prevent attacks from occurring. These medications may be given by mouth, or they may be inhaled. If an attack does occur, it is usually treated with inhaled medications (Fig. 8-9).

Chronic obstructive pulmonary disease (COPD)

Chronic obstructive pulmonary disease (COPD) takes two forms, emphysema and chronic bronchitis.

Emphysema

Emphysema is a form of COPD that involves damage to the alveoli. When a toxin, such as tobacco smoke, is inhaled, it damages the thin, delicate walls of the alveoli. Over time, the damage causes the walls of the alveoli to break. Eventually,

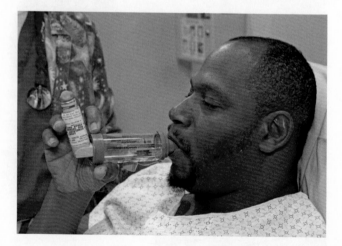

FIGURE ■ 8-9

Asthma medications are often delivered through inhalers.

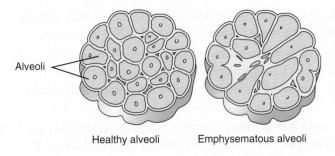

Alveoli

Healthy alveoli   Emphysematous alveoli

FIGURE ■ 8-10

A healthy lung contains millions of tiny alveoli, where gas exchange takes place. In a person with emphysema, the walls of the alveoli break down, forming large areas where air can get trapped.

Chronic bronchitis ■■■ a disorder caused by long-term irritation of the bronchi and bronchioles, such as that caused by inhaling tobacco smoke; one of two forms of chronic obstructive pulmonary disease (COPD)

instead of having millions of tiny alveoli where gas exchange can take place, the person has fewer, large "merged" alveoli (Fig. 8-10). Because the lung tissue is damaged, it is no longer "springy," and the air gets trapped in the large, damaged alveoli. The trapped air cannot be exhaled and exchanged for new oxygen-rich air, which limits the amount of oxygen the lungs are able to supply to the body. In addition, excess fluid can collect in the damaged alveoli, putting the person at risk for infection.

A person with emphysema has trouble getting a "proper breath." The person's breathing is shallow and rapid, and the person may have to stop to catch his breath quite frequently when talking or engaging in any type of physical activity. The person's chest may be enlarged and rounded ("barrel chest"). As the person's emphysema gets worse, he will need supplemental oxygen just to carry out even the simplest activities of daily living (ADLs).

Chronic bronchitis

In chronic bronchitis ongoing irritation of the bronchi leads to the production of thick mucus, which blocks the flow of air through the airways. In addition, germs can collect in the mucus, leading to infection.

A person with chronic bronchitis has a nagging, productive cough. The person may complain of "tightness" in her chest or difficulty breathing. She is likely to have frequent respiratory tract infections. Like a person with emphysema, a person with chronic bronchitis will eventually need oxygen therapy.

Cancer

In the United States, cancers involving the lungs and airway are the most common cause of cancer-related death in both men and women. Cancers that affect the respiratory system include tumors of the mouth, tongue, larynx, pharynx, bronchi, and lungs. People who smoke cigarettes are 10 times more likely to develop lung cancer than nonsmokers are. In addition, some cancers that begin in other body parts, such as the breast or intestines, commonly spread to the lungs.

Putting it all together!

■ Pneumonia, bronchitis, and influenza are common infections of the respiratory system. If untreated, these infections can be life threatening for an elderly person.

People who have chronic conditions of the respiratory system, such as asthma or COPD, may call you to the room frequently to ask for seemingly trivial things. Although this can be annoying, think about how you would feel if you had trouble breathing. Instead of giving in to the desire to avoid a "needy" patient or resident, understand the underlying fears the person may have. Spend more time with the person, and get into the habit of stopping by to check on him even when he has not called you. By addressing the person's underlying need for safety and security, you will be providing truly humanistic care.

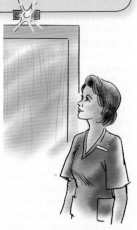

- There are two forms of chronic obstructive pulmonary disease (COPD), emphysema and chronic bronchitis. The most common cause of COPD is smoking.

- Disorders of the respiratory system can make breathing very difficult. Not being able to breathe easily can be frightening for the patient or resident. Nursing assistants provide humanistic care by helping the person to feel safe and secure.

- When caring for a person with a respiratory disorder, nursing assistants may be asked to obtain a sputum specimen for analysis. Other responsibilities of the nursing assistant when caring for a person with a respiratory disorder include observing the person for signs that he is having trouble breathing and promoting comfort.

CARDIOVASCULAR DISORDERS

What will you learn?

When you are finished with this section, you will be able to:

1. Describe two types of disorders that can affect the blood vessels.
2. Describe risk factors for developing heart disease.
3. Describe how coronary artery disease can lead to angina pectoris, myocardial infarction, or both.
4. List the signs and symptoms of a myocardial infarction ("heart attack").
5. Describe how a pacemaker is used to help a person with heart block.
6. Define the words atherosclerosis, plaque, embolus, arteriosclerosis, angina pectoris, myocardial infarction, and heart failure.

Blood vessel disorders

Atherosclerosis

Atherosclerosis ▪▪▪ blocking of the arteries, caused by the build-up of fatty deposits called plaque on the inside of the vessel wall

Plaque ▪▪▪ fatty deposits that build up on the inside of the artery wall, blocking blood flow to the tissues and making the artery wall brittle and prone to breaking

Embolus ▪▪▪ a blood clot in a vessel that breaks off and moves from one place to another

Arteriosclerosis ▪▪▪ "hardening of the arteries"; occurs when atherosclerotic plaque interferes with the elasticity of the arterial walls, making them brittle and prone to breaking

In **atherosclerosis**, **plaque** builds up on the inside of the vessél wall, blocking the flow of blood through the artery (Fig. 8-11). As a result, less oxygen and nutrients are delivered to the tissues. In addition, the plaque makes the normally smooth inner lining of the artery rough, which can cause blood clots to form. Sometimes a clot breaks off and becomes an **embolus**, which may be life threatening. The plaque also interferes with the elasticity of the arterial walls, leading to **arteriosclerosis**.

FIGURE ▪ 8-11

In atherosclerosis, fatty plaque builds up on the inside of the arteries, blocking the free flow of blood. This is particularly dangerous when the artery supplies a vital organ such as the heart, brain, or kidneys.

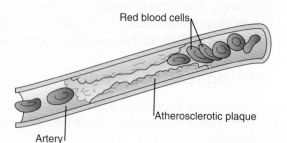

Red blood cells

Atherosclerotic plaque

Artery